THE CBT COMPANION

CBT-based models and worksheets
for practitioners and clients

THE CBT COMPANION

CBT-based models and worksheets
for practitioners and clients

BENJAMIN E. COOK

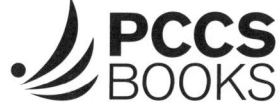

Published 2022

PCCS Books Ltd, Wyastone Business Park, Wyastone Leys, Monmouth NP25 3SR
contact@pccs-books.co.uk
www.pccs-books.co.uk

© Benjamin E. Cook, 2022

All rights reserved.
No part of this publication may be reproduced, stored in a retrieval system, transmitted or utilised in any form by any means, electronic, mechanical, photocopying (except for the blank worksheets in Appendix 2) or recording or otherwise, without permission in writing from the publishers.

The author has asserted their right to be identified as the author of this work in accordance with the Copyright, Designs and Patents Act 1988.

The CBT Companion
CBT-based models and worksheets for practitioners and clients

British Library Cataloguing in Publication data: a catalogue record for this book is available from the British Library.

ISBN   978 1 915220 18 9

Cover design Jason Anscomb
Printed in the UK by Bell & Bain Ltd, Glasgow

Contents

	About the author	*viii*
	Introduction	*1*
1	**Formulations**	**4**
1.1	Cognitive maintenance model	6
1.2	Cognitive model of panic	8
1.3	Cognitive model of perfectionism	10
1.4	Cognitive model of obsessive-compulsive disorder	12
1.5	Cognitive model of trauma	14
1.6	Vicious flowers for health anxiety	16
1.7	TRAP and TRAC	18
1.8	Chain analysis	20
1.9	ABC analysis for behavioural modification	22
1.10	Problem development model	24
1.11	Coping strategies model	26
1.12	Biopsychosocial model of health	28
2	**Goals and behavioural planning**	**30**
2.1	SMART goals	32
2.2	Nine pillars	34
2.3	Sleep hygiene checklist	36
2.4	Reality vs expectations	38
2.5	Stress quadrant	40
2.6	Phobia ladder	42
2.7	Behavioural diary	44
2.8	Identifying activities	46
2.9	Alternative solutions model	48
2.10	Exploring values	50
2.11	Value compass	52

3	**Relaxation**	**54**
3.1	Square breathing technique	56
3.2	Visual imagery	58
3.3	Progressive muscle relaxation	60
3.4	Body scan	62
3.5	Mundane task focusing	64
3.6	Grounding	66
4	**Diary-keeping**	**68**
4.1	Worry diary	70
4.2	Problematic behaviour diary	72
4.3	Relaxation diary	74
4.4	Food journal	76
4.5	Panic diary	78
4.6	Health anxiety thought record	80
4.7	Critical voice record	82
4.8	Intrusive thoughts diary	84
4.9	OCD ritual diary	86
4.10	PTSD diary	88
5	**Cognitive restructuring**	**90**
5.1	Unhelpful thinking styles	92
5.2	Thought-disputing model	94
5.3	Decatastrophising model	96
5.4	Cost/benefit analysis	98
5.5	Worry tree	100
5.6	Theory A/B model	102
5.7	Health anxiety change model	104
5.8	Core belief challenging	106
5.9	Evidence table for core beliefs	108
5.10	Cycle of beliefs, rules and behaviours	110
5.11	Rules into values	112
6	**Experiments**	**114**
6.1	Behavioural experiment	116
6.2	Resilience-developing model	118
6.3	Worry time	120

6.4	Stimulus discrimination	*122*
6.5	Imagery-based exposure	*124*
6.6	Downward arrow model	*126*
6.7	Core belief experiment	*128*
6.8	Graded exposure for phobias	*130*
6.9	OCD graded exposure	*132*
6.10	Coping cards	*134*
6.11	Cognitive cue cards	*136*
7	**Interpersonal strategies**	***138***
7.1	Acknowledging needs	*140*
7.2	Thought record for assertiveness	*142*
7.3	Assertiveness technique log	*144*
7.4	Temperature reading	*146*
7.5	Circle of contact	*148*
7.6	Responsibility pie	*150*
7.7	Cycle of abuse	*152*
8	**Relapse prevention**	***154***
8.1	Improvement and impact reflection	*156*
8.2	New coping devices reflection	*158*
8.3	Progress not perfection charts	*160*
8.4	Early warning signs	*162*
8.5	Action plan	*164*
8.6	Future plans	*166*
	Further support and resources	*168*
	Appendix 1: Thematic guides	*179*
	Appendix 2: Blank worksheets	*183*

'An artificial novelty is never as effective
as a repetition that manages to suggest a fresh truth.'

Marcel Proust
In Search of Lost Time, volume 2: Within a budding grove (1919)

About the author

Benjamin Cook is an author and practising cognitive behavioural therapist with the NHS. For the past several years he has been responsible for improving how services deliver self-guided CBT to the general public. This has involved improving access to treatment, advocating for digital therapy and working with the wider community towards reducing the stigma of mental health. Believing that therapeutic treatments need to take into account the social, economic and cultural realities of those they treat, he has constantly advocated for reflection and change on how therapy is conducted and what can be done to make therapy more inclusive. Born in the UK, he was educated at the University of St Andrews before beginning his career in East London. His practice emphasises empathy, compassion and self-realisation.

Introduction

I decided to write this book with the intention of collecting a number of therapeutic models and worksheets together in one place. This was partly as a resource for my own use and for other practitioners who might benefit from having an easily accessible reference for the tools they regularly use in treatment, but it was also for the benefit of clients. Many therapeutic modalities speak of the client becoming their own therapist but go on to make this process more difficult than it needs to be. I come from a cognitive-behavioural practice that emphasises the client, therapist and learning material as a triadic system, each a part of a collaborative exchange of ideas. So it made sense to me to make the material as clear and concise as possible for everyone concerned.

Often there is a risk of mystifying the process – how an individual experiencing mental health difficulties goes through a transformation in therapy and comes out on the other side reborn as a new person. Jargon, unnecessarily complex systems of thought and the notion of the therapist as omniscient all reinforce the idea that the client is a passive receptacle. Fortunately, in the last few decades this has changed considerably, as the proliferation of self-help books testifies. We are now much more willing to 'become our own therapist' – to see what we can do ourselves to produce change in our lives. And increasingly therapists too are actively working to enable their clients to take these steps.

Nevertheless, there are professionals who believe that the models and formulations described in this book impose an unhelpful artificiality; that they attempt to fit the diverse problems of individuals into pre-arranged patterns. If every individual's problems are unique, how can any model truly capture what it is they are experiencing? To unpack this idea, it is crucial to recognise the similarities that all humans have, while remaining conscious of not reducing a person to a collection of physical or mental symptoms.

The models and worksheets here are based on cognitive-behavioural therapy (CBT) principles. These principles involve the idea that the significance we attribute to experiences influences how we feel and behave, that unhealthy beliefs sustain maladaptive coping strategies and that it is within our power to change how we think and act. It is a therapeutic model that is structured, time limited and involves an empirical approach to testing out dysfunctional assumptions. Focus is placed on problem-solving present difficulties while coming to an understanding of how those problems might have been maintained for so long. While individuals will present with complex histories, it is possible to narrow down the most appropriate treatment options by recognising what it is they are experiencing – for example, anxiety, depression, stress and so on – and creating a customised plan around this presentation. This widely used, evidence-based treatment offers the rigour of the medical-diagnostic model while still providing enough flexibility to accommodate the uniqueness of individuals. For all these reasons, CBT encourages clients to learn from as many resources as possible, including models and worksheets.

It can be helpful to consider why therapists use models and worksheets in the first place. First, they offer insight into our difficulties. By listing our experiences, we are able to see how our problems intensify in the moment and recur time after time. They encourage reflection, and it is often only with reflection that we can see that change is needed. For instance, when we are experiencing something distressful, our attention is focused on the source of distress; we are caught up in our emotions and it is difficult to get the emotional distance to see our problems objectively. After such experiences, recollecting what we were thinking and feeling can be difficult; hence the need to write down our experiences as soon as possible in order to retain them for future reflection. This serves two purposes. It puts the responsibility on us to organise our time and energy towards the goal of improving our mental health, and it allows us later to sit back with a therapist or on our own and consider our triggers, our maintenance cycles or our unhelpful thinking styles or behaviours.

All of this highlights an important fact: change rarely comes from an epiphany or flash of insight; instead, it comes from the work we put into changing our thinking and behaviours when fully engaged in the messiness of life. You will notice as you progress through the chapters in this book that many models involve going out into the world and testing our assumptions. Nothing teaches better than experience. What has been learned unconsciously through negative experiences often needs to be relearned through managed interventions that challenge preconceived notions of the world and our place within it.

How to use this book

A brief note on how to use this book. It is organised in eight thematic chapters, each of which focuses on a number of models with accompanying worksheets. Each model starts with a reference to a published chapter, paper or article that provides the theory underpinning it. It goes on to describe what it's for, when it might be useful and for whom, and how to complete the accompanying worksheet. With each model, there is a completed worksheet, already filled out with a fictional example. At the back of the book, there are blank copies of these worksheets, which you can copy as many times as you like and complete yourself.

Speaking now to the individual reader who has picked up the challenge to 'become their own therapist', this book is not designed to be read from cover to cover; nor do I suggest you work through every worksheet in it. Some of them will simply not be relevant to your needs. The introductions that precede every worksheet should make it clear whether or not you will find any benefit from a particular exercise. You will also find suggestions under the 'suitability' headings where specific models can be paired with others. These are just recommendations, though: feel free to experiment with anything that you think might be helpful.

For those who might appreciate more structure, I have drawn up a number of thematic guides (Appendix 1), each one covering a specific difficulty: depression, generalised anxiety, stress, phobias, OCD and PTSD. You can follow these plans with clients who have a recognisable presentation; the suggested models cover many of the steps necessary to see progress.

Be wary of trying to do too much too soon; it may be overwhelming, and if you have to stop because you have taken on too many models at once, you are less likely to pick up this book again. I suggest you choose one or two models per week from a particular chapter and dedicate your time to completing them. While some worksheets can be completed in one sitting, many require you to constantly refer back to them at the end of each day and fill in the questions. At the end of the week, you can set aside some time to reflect on what you have completed and then move on the next chapter.

There are some chapters that are exceptions to this rule. The chapters on relaxation and relapse prevention can be read from start to finish and should be completed in their entirety. When you move on to another chapter, do not abandon the previous worksheets but think about how you can continue working on them and integrate them into any further learning.

By the end of eight weeks, you should start to see your problems become significantly more manageable. This should inspire you with increased confidence in your abilities. If this is the case, you may decide to put the book to one side, while continuing to integrate its lessons into your daily life. If you feel you would benefit from more support, you can revisit some of the other models that you skipped over the first time around, or you can explore the additional resources listed at the back of the book. These include mental health organisations, books and self-help apps, all of which will help reinforce the lessons contained here. If you feel that you are still struggling, consider speaking to a professional who might be able to address your difficulties with you in more depth or from another therapeutic modality. All the additional resources in this book are designed for a UK readership, but many other countries should be able to provide support that mirrors what is accessible in the UK.

Again, I say to the individual user, no matter where you are on your journey to improve your mental health, it is important to see the progress that you make in a compassionate light. One of the most difficult things about becoming your own therapist is the loss of the human element. The genuineness, empathy and understanding of a therapist is something no book can replicate, which makes it all the more critical that you identify those systems of support that you do have: your family, friends and your wider community, but also those internal strengths that might have been forgotten in recent months. Look at what you are able to accomplish here as your first steps towards realising your goals. If the first few steps are unsteady, know that the more you take, the firmer the ground beneath your feet will feel. I hope that by the end of this book you will feel more certain of yourself and your ability to face your issues head on.

And to the practitioner who is using this book to work through relevant exercises with their clients, I suggest letting your clients guide you in the choice of what models to use. When you first begin assessing a client, ask yourself what model here best captures what your client is experiencing. The purpose of the formulations in Chapter 1 are, after all, designed to help a client make sense of their difficulties, to normalise what they are experiencing and to show how they can disrupt their maintenance cycles that have developed over time. Once you have identified what you both believe to the central problem, highlight the relevant models that your professional judgement suggests might be of help. Which model does the client feel most comfortable to begin with? Which model addresses their most urgent needs?

The use of therapeutic models does not mean that you have to sacrifice a collaborative approach to therapy. One of the joys of engaging in a therapeutic relationship with another is the spirit of creativity as you together explore patterns of thought and behaviour and uncover new ways to understand how the pieces of the jigsaw fit together. You should take exactly this creative approach to using these models. At the start of the book are some 'thematic guides' that suggest how you might organise a treatment plan based on a client's presenting issues. However, it is best to think of these as templates that you can add to and adjust to fit your client's needs and preferences, not as a rigid prescription. This structured mix-and-match approach allows a degree of flexibility while still adhering to the evidence base of what works best.

My hope is that this book will provide a foundation for you to further develop your learning and practice. In order to help with this, I make suggestions for further reading for most of the models. Some are classics in CBT literature, some are academic sources, and some are simply books that build on the principles hinted at in the models themselves. In therapy, we speak of learning as a continuous process; new evidence that supports or challenges our beliefs is always accumulating. I hope this book finds a place alongside what you already know and encourages you to explore further and develop your skills.

Chapter 1. Formulations

Introduction

This chapter is concerned with understanding how mental health difficulties are maintained. Many of the formulations are based on cognitive-behavioural therapy (CBT) principles, and as such emphasise the importance of behaviour and cognitions for physical and mental health. The worksheets and diagrams that follow will explore the behaviours that we adopt as coping devices to alleviate stress and the unhelpful thinking styles that distort how we see reality.

As is common in CBT treatments, there is a great degree of specificity that separates one worksheet from another. You will see this highlighted in some of the titles, as well as under the 'suitability' headings in each individual worksheet introduction. This is derived from the medical-diagnostic worksheet, where such conditions as social anxiety, depression, phobias or PTSD are classified as individual disorders that have specific treatment plans. While many disorders share similar characteristics, there is ample evidence to suggest that a one-plan-fits-all approach is neither sufficient nor desirable in many cases. To give an example, social anxiety shares many traits with other anxiety disorders, but it also includes a heightened sense that others are constantly judging you and that you must excessively monitor your performance in social situations to ensure you make no mistakes. This suggests that, although individuals experiencing social anxiety might benefit from such generic formulations as the ABC Analysis for Behavioural Modification (p.22) or Chain Analysis (p.20), they might benefit more from specific worksheets tailored to their needs, such as the Cognitive Model of Panic (p.8). By introducing this level of specificity, you can pick and choose the formulations that best reflect what the client is currently experiencing.

Regardless of the type or severity of their condition, it is suggested that the client begins with the Cognitive Maintenance Model (p.6), as it provides an excellent introduction to understanding how problems are reinforced by our behaviours and thoughts. An understanding of the worksheet will allow you to explore more complex worksheets with your client, such as the Cognitive Model of Trauma (p.14) or the Cognitive Model of Obsessive-Compulsive Disorder (p.12), which apply a similar philosophy but go into more detail regarding the role of attention and catastrophic thinking.

As you delve into this chapter, you will notice that there are a few worksheets that go beyond the idea that our problems are maintained by our thoughts and behaviours to include other factors, such as our environment, history and inherent vulnerabilities. This is to highlight how the psychological sits beside social and genetic factors as reasons for why difficulties arise and why we are resistant to change. While this book will focus on what is well within our power to change, it is important to stress that our responsibility for the severity of our problems is often much less than we might assume. The Biopsychosocial Model of Health (p.28) attempts to open up the possibility that, while our thoughts and behaviours might be maintaining our problems, it is possible that they did not originate from them.

Ultimately, any insight into how our problems are maintained needs to highlight why our own behaviours and thoughts are conspiring against us to make our life miserable. This can occasionally be a difficult thing to acknowledge, as it seems to run contrary to common sense. Why would anybody act constantly against their own self-interest? TRAP and TRAC (p.18) does the heavy lifting here and tries to communicate how we will prioritise short-term relief at the cost of long-term benefit. We are by our very nature problem-solvers, but occasionally we adopt solutions that are not as effective as we initially assume. These thoughts can be further explored in Problem Development Model (p.24) and Coping Strategies Model (p.26), which both look at the quality of our coping skills and invite opportunities for change.

I invite you to use the following formulations and maintenance cycles to clarify what it is that you or your client is facing and what is within your control to change. While it might be tempting to avoid our triggers or isolate ourselves from others, often these solutions will make us feel worse, not better. Awareness of these shortcomings is sometimes enough to produce change, and later chapters will explore what further resources we have at our disposal to overcome difficulties.

1.1 Cognitive Maintenance Model

Padesky, C.A. & Mooney, K.A. (1990). Clinical tip: Presenting the cognitive model to clients. *International Cognitive Therapy Newsletter*, *6*, 13–14.

Purpose

The first stage to understanding why an emotion can be so intense is to see it as part of an intricate but intuitive system. The Cognitive Maintenance Model is designed to highlight how our emotions do not simply appear on their own but are, in fact, triggered by specific situations and then reinforced by our thoughts, behaviour and physical symptoms. For instance, the level of frustration that we feel at hearing bad news can be increased or decreased by the significance we attribute to that news. What meaning do we give the news, and do we see it as saying something about us? If so, does that have an impact on how we view the world and behave with others?

In a similar manner, our physical symptoms can influence how we feel. If the bad news is given to us when we are already feeling tired and low, it is more than likely that our emotions will be stronger. Strong emotional reactions can also then lead to further physical symptoms appearing, which can range from a flushed face to a full-on panic attack.

When we are experiencing all these negative symptoms and thoughts, we will often respond by changing our behaviour to cope with and remove those unpleasant sensations. The model circles back on itself in this respect, as it aims to distinguish between those coping devices that have long-term positive consequences and those that only offer short-term relief. Often it is the adoption of inappropriate or maladaptive coping strategies that can lead over time to significant mental health difficulties.

Suitability

The model is suitable for anyone trying to learn more about CBT principles and is recommended as a gentle introduction before you move on to other, more specific maintenance models. This model can be used throughout treatment as a way to highlight any additional difficulties that have surfaced since the start of your journey to improve your mental health.

How to use

If you are unsure what experiences should be recorded, start by recalling those times when your emotions were particularly heightened and then work backwards from there, identifying in as much detail as possible the situation you found yourself in. Ask yourself:

- Who was I with?
- What was the time?
- Where was I?

Once you have grounded the emotions in a specific time and place, it is usually easier to recall the thoughts and physical symptoms that occurred alongside them.

It is a good idea to record as much as you can, especially with the thoughts. Often, once a number of these models have been completed, a pattern of recurring negative thoughts will emerge, and these can be a springboard for further investigation. Finish by recording the behaviour that you were engaged in when the emotions were at their most intense and what you did to reduce that intensity. This is a great opportunity to reflect on whether you think your coping devices are adequate or if they need improvement.

When everything has been completed, take an overall look at the finished model and note how each symptom is related to the others. The more versions of this model you complete, the easier it becomes to comprehend how frequently one symptom links to another.

Formulations 7

Cognitive Maintenance Model

Specific situation

My boss just told me that they will have to cut my working hours

Thoughts

What am I going to do without that extra money?

They should have given me more warning. How dare they treat me like this

I'm no good at anything

Physical symptoms

Flushed face

Headache

Tiredness

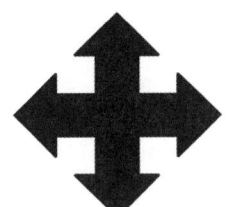

Emotions

Sad

Dejected

Angry

Frustrated

Behaviours/coping devices

Avoided sharing the news with my family

Spent more time during the weekend alone

Stayed silent when my boss broke the news

1.2 Cognitive Model of Panic

Clark, D.M. (1986). A cognitive approach to panic. *Behaviour Research and Therapy, 24*, 461–70.

Purpose

The Cognitive Model of Panic explains how panic attacks begin and are maintained by our thoughts and how we interpret our physical symptoms. A panic attack will involve several physical symptoms, such as:

- chest pain or discomfort
- chills or hot sensations
- feeling of choking
- feeling dizzy, unsteady, lightheaded or faint
- fear of dying
- fear of losing control or going crazy
- feelings of unreality.

These symptoms are often misinterpreted as being more dangerous than they actually are. In reality, the symptoms usually last for only a few minutes and cause us no lasting harm. But they can be incredibly distressing to experience – you can feel as though you are about to have a heart attack, and people often reach for extreme coping devices, such as calling for an ambulance.

Suitability

People experiencing panic attacks or panic disorder should find this model particularly helpful in understanding situational triggers and the role of catastrophic misinterpretation in increasing their symptoms. It is a good introduction to exploring how panic is maintained and how it can be managed by refocusing attention elsewhere.

How to use

This model distinguishes between two triggers: internal and external. Many panic attacks are caused by exposure to anxiety-inducing situations. These can be specific external threats that are misinterpreted to be more dangerous than they are. Agoraphobia (fear of open spaces) is a good example of an external trigger that can lead to panic attacks.

Internal triggers can cause panic attacks seemingly from nowhere. In reality, these panic attacks come from too great a focus on your body or on your breathing. If, for example, you are running to catch a bus, the consequent increase in heart rate, breathing and light-headedness, which are signs of physical exertion, can be misinterpreted as something more ominous. As your anxiety increases, so do the physical symptoms, effectively maintaining them at levels beyond those the physical effort would warrant. If this happens often, it is possible that you are experiencing symptoms of a panic disorder.

In many cases, a mixture of external and internal triggers causes thoughts that greatly exaggerate a perceived threat. These thoughts are then reinforced by physical symptoms, emotions and the specific unhelpful thinking style of catastrophic misinterpretation. When listing these aspects of your panic attack, be sure to give thought to how each might influence the other and so escalate the length and intensity of your panic.

Cognitive Model of Panic

Internal trigger

Struggling to catch my breath

Elevated heart rate

External trigger

Running to catch a bus

Trying to find my money to pay for the bus

Perceived threat

I can't breathe. I might pass out

Emotion

Fear

Nervousness

Catastrophic misinterpretation

I am going to have a heart attack

Physical symptoms

Dizziness

Shaking

Sweating

1.3 The Cognitive Model of Perfectionism

Shafran, R., Egan, S. & Wade, T. (2018). *Overcoming perfectionism: A self-help guide using cognitive behavioural techniques*. Robinson.

Purpose

Perfectionism can be understood as holding yourself to a higher standard than you expect of others, to such an extent that it has a detrimental effect on your life. It is often more complex than simply wanting things to be perfect. In many cases, it involves deep-seated core beliefs about self-worth and how you value your own efforts.

Perfectionist habits and thoughts can be easily maintained as they are often mistakenly conflated with more positive beliefs about ambition, good performance and productivity. It can be easy to argue that to give up perfectionism would be to give up on these other beliefs, but that is not necessarily the case. When you challenge perfectionism, you are challenging the idea that your self-worth is entirely based on reaching certain rigid standards – standards that, in many cases, are unrealistic and set you up to fail.

The Cognitive Model of Perfectionism is intended to demonstrate the above principles and explain the cycle that maintains and reinforces perfectionist behaviours and thoughts. It also helps highlight how selective information processing keeps perfectionism in place. If, for example, you judge yourself based on your performance, it is more than likely that you will give greater significance to your imperfections while neglecting the aspects that are successful, and so increase your emotional distress and further reduce your sense of self-worth.

Suitability

This model is useful for anyone who wants to explore their perfectionist beliefs or behaviours. If you are experiencing a great degree of stress, it is worth asking whether that is due to specific perfectionist ways of looking at situations. Similarly, if you have low self-esteem, could that be caused by a discrepancy in how you judge yourself in comparison with how you judge others? As this model touches on core beliefs and rules, I generally suggest it is used alongside the material on cognitive restructuring in Chapter 5.

How to use

I suggest you begin by identifying what your unrelenting standard is. If there are several, use additional copies of the worksheet so that your perfectionist behaviours and thoughts do not get entangled. Try to list several thoughts and behaviours that you think might be the result of holding an unrelenting standard. Then, drawing on past situations, complete as best you can the consequences of reaching and failing to reach that unrelenting standard.

If you believe you fail to meet your unrelenting standards, the arrows on the worksheet indicate you should ask yourself what, in very general terms, you base your sense of self-worth on and what rules you need to put in place to reach that ideal. The phrases 'I should...' and 'I must...' will help highlight the inflexibility of the demands that you put on yourself and the need to change.

If you are able to meet your standards, follow the arrow back to the unrelenting standard and imagine how doing so might change it. Could you rest on your success? Or would you need to raise your standards further and push yourself harder? The aim here is to show you how perfectionism traps you in a bind of never-ending failure, no matter how hard you try.

Cognitive Model of Perfectionism

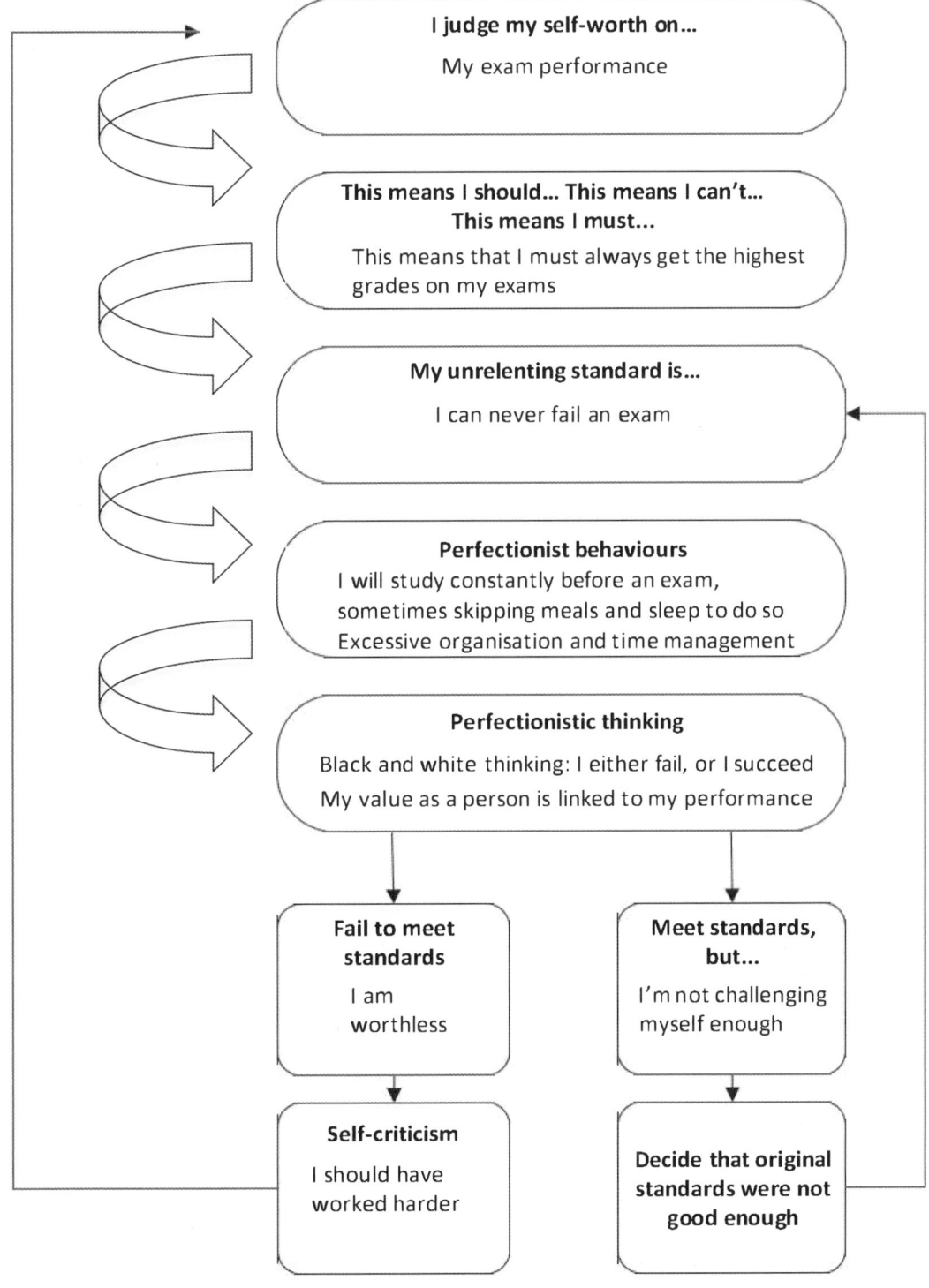

1.4 Cognitive Model of Obsessive-Compulsive Disorder

Salkovskis, P.M., Forrester, E., & Richards, C. (1998). Cognitive-behavioural approach to understanding obsessional thinking. *British Journal of Psychiatry, 173*(S35), 53–63.

Purpose

Obsessive-compulsive disorder (OCD) is characterised by repetitive, intrusive thoughts about impending catastrophe and the resulting behaviours that attempt to neutralise or reduce those thoughts. These thoughts/obsessions bring on an intense sense of anxiety about the anticipated catastrophe that can only be allayed by carrying out a specific activity or ritual, such as washing hands, checking light switches, praying and so forth, thoroughly enough to avert it. In reality, the compulsive behaviour will only reduce the anxiety, at best; it cannot influence any real-world disaster. Despite this evident lack of causative power, OCD can be very difficult to overcome. You might be able to see that your actions are not entirely rational but still be powerless to stop them.

One of the reasons that OCD is maintained over time is that, every time you act on your obsessions by performing the compulsive behaviours and the catastrophic outcome you feared doesn't happen, you chalk that up to having performed those compulsive behaviours. This is an unhelpful thinking style sometimes referred to as magical thinking – you believe that your actions have a profound but unjustified influence on events around you. If you believe that only you can save your family from being poisoned by a gas leak, your compulsive checking to make sure the gas is switched off no longer seems entirely irrational.

The Cognitive Model of Obsessive-Compulsive Disorder explores how these intrusive thoughts are strengthened by the meanings that we attribute to them, to our avoidance of certain actions and to the repetitive behaviours that we do to neutralise our obsessive beliefs. All of these combine to ensure that the cycle of OCD remains intact and harmful to our mental wellbeing.

Suitability

The Cognitive Model of Obsessive-Compulsive Disorder is a good first step for you if you want to understand more about your obsessions and compulsive behaviours. It pairs well with the Intrusive Thoughts Diary (Chapter 4, p.84) and the OCD Graded Exposure worksheet (Chapter 6, p.132).

How to use

Start by identifying a past intrusive thought and then describe the triggering situation you were in. Describe the place, any people you were with and the time. Then ask yourself what meaning you gave the thought and what that says about you and your perceptions of the world. Once you have come to some conclusions, you might be better able to see how and why it caused such strong emotions. Often the core beliefs you uncover can be very self-critical or disclose an unsettling way of seeing the world.

Go on to explore what you next did in reaction to the thought. Did you avoid anything, or did you act out one of your compulsions? Did your attempt to neutralise the intrusive thought work? If it did, what does that tell you about the compulsive behaviour? These questions can lead you to a better understanding of how compulsions can reinforce the fear either of the situation or of the intrusive thought itself. This is because the more effective we believe our compulsions to be, the harder it is for us to let them go and replace them with more helpful and coping devices.

Cognitive Model of Obsessive-Compulsive Disorder

Trigger

Finished cooking a meal for my family on our gas stove

Intrusive thought

If I don't turn off the gas properly, I could set the house on fire

Avoidance, emotional response and neutralisation reinforce fear of trigger and fear of the intrusive thought

Emotions

Fear
Panic
Doubt

Meaning of intrusive thought

I am entirely responsible for my family's safety

Avoidance

Reduce using the gas stove

Ask my partner to do the cooking

Neutralisation

When using the gas stove, I make sure to check several times that I have turned it off properly

1.5 The Cognitive Model of Trauma

Ehlers, A. & Clark, D.M. (2000). A cognitive model of posttraumatic stress disorder. *Behaviour Research and Therapy, 38*, 319–345.

Purpose

Not every traumatic life event leads to symptoms of post-traumatic stress disorder (PTSD), but when it happens, it can be a bewildering and frightening experience. Common signs that you may be experiencing PTSD are recurring flashbacks and nightmares, emotional numbing, dissociation and hyperarousal. Often these symptoms can combine with harmful coping devices such as alcohol dependency, drug misuse or social withdrawal, as the person does their best to avoid situations that trigger their traumatic memories.

When, for instance, flashbacks occur, the past and the present blur and it can feel as if you are reliving those traumatic memories all over again. It is because of the immediacy of the memory that we go to such lengths to avoid them recurring, but these efforts often prove futile. The Cognitive Model of Trauma is designed to reverse avoidance by helping us to confront those memories so that, eventually, the difference between what belongs to the past and what is in the present becomes clearer.

This model looks at how the memories of the traumatic event are influenced and shaped by our beliefs about the world and self. If we hold the belief that the world is a dangerous place and we are then harmed, that belief is going to become much stronger. If those beliefs become stronger, we are more likely to take increasingly drastic measures to keep ourselves safe. If no further traumatising event occurs, we will attribute that to our maladaptive coping strategies and not to any radical change in our current situation.

Suitability

The model is suitable for people who are experiencing symptoms of trauma. As revisiting traumatic memories can be distressing, it is worth enlisting the help of a therapist to guide you through this process. If that is not possible, make sure that you complete this model in a place where you feel safe. I suggest you master the Grounding relaxation technique (Chapter 3, p.66) before attempting this model.

How to use

Start by naming the traumatic event you want to explore. This can be difficult and upsetting in itself. Be sure to ground yourself in the present and remind yourself to be self-compassionate. Once you have named the traumatic event, list the memories that resurface. It can be helpful to use your senses as a prompt: What did you hear then? What did you see then? and so forth. By doing this, you can paint a picture of the trauma that is true to your experience of it.

Now imagine the most recent time you felt threatened – for example, when you became hyperaroused and overly conscious of potential threat or you felt yourself disconnect from the here and now. When that feeling of being in danger overtook you, how did you respond and what actions did you take to alleviate it? Remember, even if you took no overt physical action, your response can be worth investigating. Did you run to find safety, seize something to defend yourself, or freeze and hope the danger would pass on its own?

The final section is about your beliefs about the world and your place within it. These beliefs may be ones you held before the traumatic event, or they may have developed afterwards. As long as you can see some tangential connection to how you might be feeling now, they are worth noting. Often these beliefs can revolve around a sense of personal vulnerability or of the world not being a safe place. If that is the case, think about how your coping strategies weaken or strengthen those beliefs.

Formulations 15

Cognitive Model of Trauma

Traumatic event

Being assaulted when in a nightclub

Memories of the trauma

The taste of blood in my mouth

All the screaming that was going on during the assault

Beliefs about the world and my place in it...

I am only safe when I am travelling in groups

The world is an inherently dangerous place

CURRENT SENSE OF THREAT

Coping strategies

I avoid going to nightclubs

I only leave the house at night when I am with others

When I am anxious, I call my family for reassurance

1.6 Vicious Flowers for Health Anxiety

Salkovskis, P.M. & Warwick, H. (2001). Making sense of hypochondriasis: A cognitive theory of health anxiety. In G. Asmundson, S. Taylor & B.J. Cox (Eds.), *Health anxiety: Clinical and research perspectives on hypochondriasis and related conditions* (pp 46–64). Wiley.

Purpose

Health anxiety is the persistent worry that you will become ill or that your health will very shortly and rapidly deteriorate. Like other types of anxiety, it is strengthened by an intolerance of uncertainty, which can make small, otherwise trivial physical symptoms seem like a precursor to something much worse. It is not uncommon for someone with health anxiety to have an actual health condition. This can be a genuine worry, but a tell-tale sign of health anxiety is the maintenance of excessive worry through specific unhelpful thinking styles and checking and reassurance behaviours. These coping strategies might reduce the anxiety in the short term, but in the long term they encourage the idea that constant vigilance towards your body is the only way to stay safe.

By focusing attention on your body, you become much more attuned to any inner shifts or disturbances that occur regularly throughout the day. Only now you attribute these changes to a serious underlying health condition, instead of to your body's natural rhythms. Obviously, this will increase anxiety. When anxiety increases to a certain level, so too will a number of physical symptoms, such as heart palpitations, shaking, headaches and so on. These additional symptoms can then be worked into your narrative that something is terribly wrong with your health. After all, why else would you be feeling this way?

Vicious Flowers for Health Anxiety is designed to help you recognise the behaviours and thoughts that perpetuate excessive worry. Common behaviours can be constantly seeking reassurance about your health from family and friends, constantly making appointments with your doctor for reassessment, and avoiding physical activities in case they exacerbate your symptoms. Common beliefs can be that you need to constantly check your health for changes, that doctors are incompetent and that you need to research the causes of any newly discovered physical symptoms on the internet.

Suitability

The model can be useful to anyone who experiences anxiety about their health, but it will work most effectively with people who recognise themselves in the descriptions above. Health anxiety is often maintained by selective attention to the body. If you have noticed that, when you feel physical discomfort, you start to examine your body for confirmation of your beliefs about your health, you will find this model an appropriate introduction to reducing the anxiety that results from such checking behaviour.

How to use

Start by writing your health worry at the centre of the model. This can be a precise physical symptom or it can be an illness that you have or believe yourself to have. Next, figure out what behaviours and thoughts might be maintaining this worry. You may think they are necessary to keep you safe, but you should still note them down. The aim of this model is not to challenge your actions and beliefs but to come to an understanding of how they might be maintaining the worry. Any challenging can be done later, if needed, using other models.

Once you have completed the model, ask yourself what you could change that might have a positive effect on how you feel. Even if you are not willing to confront the fact that anxiety might be the source of your discomfort, it is often possible to see that certain behaviours and thoughts are unproductive, and this in itself can be the first step towards meaningful change.

Vicious Flowers for Health Anxiety

There is something wrong with my body...
I am experiencing irritable bowel syndrome (IBS)

Maintaining factor
I avoid public places without access to toilets

Maintaining factor
I worry that I will have to live with this forever

Maintaining factor
I contact my GP regularly whenever a new symptom presents itself

Maintaining factor
I am constantly embarrassed when I discuss my health issues with friends/family

Maintaining factor
I am constantly revising my diet to look for foods that don't trigger the IBS

Maintaining factor
I am constantly researching my condition on the internet

Maintaining factor
I do not trust the professional advice I receive, as so far it has not been helpful to me

Maintaining factor
I avoid social outings in restaurants where I might need to eat unfamiliar food

1.7 TRAP and TRAC

Martell, C.R., Addis, M.E. & Jacobson, N.S. (2001). *Depression in context: Strategies for guided action.* W.W. Norton & Co.

Purpose

When we act in haste or from heightened emotions, we rarely have time to think through the consequences of our actions. The short-term relief of distress is emphasised over the long-term consequences of our avoidance behaviour. This is quite natural. If we feel terrible, our first course of action is usually to remove or get away from whatever it is that makes us feel that way. Ultimately, all that matters in the short term is that our distress reduces. We will grab with both hands any solution that achieves that end.

Unfortunately, what improves the mood in the short term can lead to unforeseen consequences in the long term. If, for example, you respond to an unpleasant social interaction by isolating yourself from social contact, you will succeed in reducing your current anxiety. That short burst of relief when you leave a social situation will motivate you to do it again and again. The long-term consequences of this isolation might not be apparent straight away. It may even provide some respite for a short while, as you focus on yourself without distraction. Nevertheless, in time, repeatedly isolating yourself when you feel any anxiety or discomfort could lead to those positive social relationships falling apart. Loneliness might follow, and then self-recrimination.

TRAP and TRAC allows you to take a closer look at the consequences of your actions. It is possible that many avoidance behaviours could be transformed into alternative coping strategies, which simply means that the long-term consequences of your actions become more aligned with your goals. You avoid the traps and get back on track!

Suitability

TRAP and TRAC provides insight to anybody looking to test out the long-term usefulness of their coping strategies. While the maintenance cycle is useful on its own, the model's primary strength lies in how it illustrates the long-term repercussions of your behaviours and presents opportunities to contemplate change. This model works particularly well with the goal-oriented material in Chapter 2.

How to use

Start by filling in the TRAP worksheet. Focus on a specific situation in your recent past that caused you distress and work your way through the model, paying close attention to any avoidance behaviours you took. Once you have recorded what happened, try to remember what the consequences were at the time or in the following days. Then imagine what the long-term consequences would be if you acted that way every time you found yourself in a similar situation.

Next, move on to the TRAC worksheet. Fill out the trigger and the thoughts/feelings for the same situation you just covered with the TRAP worksheet, only this time try to imagine what would have happened if you had acted differently. Picture yourself responding with the benefit of hindsight and write down your alternative coping strategy. Finish by imagining the alternative consequences, both short- and long-term. You might find the short-term consequences are more unpleasant than those you identified for TRAP, but hopefully the long-term consequences will be significantly more positive and encourage a change of direction.

TRAP worksheet

Trigger	**R**esponse	**A**voidance **P**attern
Event	Thoughts/feelings	Specific examples of behaviour that reduces the intensity of thoughts and feelings
I was in town and I saw my friend on the opposite side of the street. I called out to her but she didn't pay any attention and kept on walking	I thought she had ignored me on purpose I tried to think of what I could have done that would have offended her I felt hurt I was embarrassed as I had shouted in public	I decided to not go to a party that she was having at the weekend I blocked her on my phone
Short-term consequences		Long-term consequences
I did not go to her party I spent the weekend at home and didn't go out much I avoided checking social media I spent the next few days thinking about the incident		I damaged our friendship when she found out I had blocked her on my phone It has made me more hesitant about going to social occasions where I might be ignored I now feel more lonely

TRAC worksheet

Trigger	**R**esponse	**A**lternative **C**oping
Event	Thoughts/feelings	Specific examples of behaviour that reduces the intensity of thoughts and feelings
I was in town and I saw my friend on the opposite side of the street. I called out to her but she didn't pay any attention and kept on walking.	I thought she had ignored me on purpose I tried to think of what I could have done that would have offended her I was embarrassed as I had shouted in public I was a little angry as there was no justification for snubbing me	I gave my friend a call later that day and told her I had seen her in town. She apologised for being distracted and told me she had been going through a lot lately. We made plans to talk more at her party.
Short-term consequences		Long-term consequences
Anxiety over calling my friend and confronting her about not responding to me Went to friend's party and had a good time Managed to speak to my friend at the party and she told me about the death of a relative. I expressed my sympathy and sadness for her		Got closer to my friend Made new friends at the party Became more confident to express my concerns to friends

1.8 Chain Analysis

Rizvi, S.L. & Ritschel, L.A. (2014). Mastering the art of Chain Analysis in dialectical behavior therapy. *Cognitive and Behavioral Practice*, *21*(3), 335–349.

Purpose

Chain Analysis targets behaviours that we wish we could stop. It reveals the sequence whereby a triggering situation leads to an array of emotions, behaviours and thoughts that eventually culminate in the unwanted behaviour. The more we can understand that process, the easier it is to put a stop to it.

The image of a chain is particularly resonant, as we are often held fast by our thoughts and behaviours and can struggle to regain freedom. A chain, too, is never simply one link; rather, it is a long sequence that wraps itself around us and refuses to let go. It is necessary to be able to identify the habitual sequences that trigger our unwanted behaviour, but it is important also to be able to see which rings of the chain can be broken and swapped out. How do we make a new sequence that does not bind us to the same mistakes of the old one?

There is no simple answer to this, as all the other models in this book also testify. It can take time to learn the different strategies – whether it is cognitive restructuring, mindfulness or simply disengaging from conflict. That said, it is possible to frustrate the consistency of unwanted behaviours by implementing small changes that, over time, can have a significant impact on our coping abilities.

Suitability

Chain Analysis can be used to target any specific behaviour that you wish to change. It is relevant to anyone who has found their recent behaviour to be counterproductive. For example, people who self-harm or practise self-destructive behaviours might find it helps to track the sequence from a trigger to the behaviour. Later in treatment, the model can be used to refine the therapeutic and non-therapeutic strategies we have learned through psychoeducation and use in our daily interactions.

How to use

Start by identifying a behaviour that you wish to change. Next, ask yourself what precursors could have made you more susceptible to this behaviour. These precursors can be anything that you believe has relevance. Then move on to describe the usual trigger that brings on the unwanted behaviour.

Next, complete the chain of events, physical symptoms, emotional reactions, unhelpful thoughts and so forth that lead to the unwanted behaviour. It can be difficult to decide the order of the rings in the chain – does the headache come before or after the thought that you are a failure? Ultimately, the order is not important. What matters is that you have tracked a sequence that explains why a particular trigger consistently causes the same unwanted outcome.

Finally, on the far right of the model, identify the rings of the chain that can be changed. Small behaviours are often a good place to start. A change in your posture or the tone of your voice can make a difference to how you feel, which in turn might let you be more compassionate towards yourself and others. If you swapped out your usual sequence for this new one, what would be the outcome? Would it be the same unwanted behaviour or would something have changed?

Formulations 21

	Usual sequence	New sequence
Target behaviour to change When I get upset, I lose control and cry	I think to myself, I haven't planned for this, what will I do?	I accept that uncertainty is a part of life
Precursors I have always had difficulty with controlling my emotions	I feel overwhelmed, as if the world is collapsing in on me	I focus on previous times when I have successfully overcome challenges
	I start to move and speak really quickly	I sit down and slow down my speech.
Trigger When something unexpected occurs	I worry that I will not be able to foresee all the things that will go wrong	I identify my catastrophising thought and find competing evidence against it

Chain Analysis

	I start to shake	I practise specific relaxation exercises
	I have to get away from people	I refocus my attention on others and engage with the present

Usual outcome	New outcome
I break down in tears	I successfully control my emotional reactions

1.9 ABC Analysis for Behavioural Modification

Tarrier, N. & Calam, R. (2002). New developments in cognitive-behavioural case formulation. *Behavioural and Cognitive Psychotherapy*, *30*, 311–328.

Purpose

The consequences of our behaviour can often lead to unhappy situations. Yet, to change behaviour, it is first necessary to identify what causes it and the consequences that follow. ABC Analysis for Behavioural Modification clarifies the triggering situation, the maladaptive behaviours that follow and the consequences of your actions, thereby allowing you to see where you might make meaningful change.

These possible interventions can occur at the antecedent level, where you plan in advance how to avoid or intervene early to de-escalate triggering situations; at the behavioural level, where you respond in a different way, and at the consequence level, where you prevent your behaviour from causing any further distress. By separating these three components, it becomes easier to see where modifications can be made. Often it can seem as though unhelpful behaviours come from nowhere and, once enacted, have consequences that you cannot avoid. In fact, as the model shows, there are always many ways to prevent what seems to be the inevitable.

Suitability

This model can be used to target maladaptive behaviours and so would be helpful if you wanted to identify the antecedents that bring them on and the consequences that follow. The identification of potential interventions makes this model useful if you want to see immediate opportunities for change.

How to use

Start by focusing on a recent behaviour that was unhelpful. It might be one specific behaviour or there might be several aspects or tangents that are worth recording. Then list under 'Antecedents' the triggers that brought on this behaviour. They can be factors that happened directly before the behaviour, but they can also include context detail, such as your mood that day or your sleep the night before. Provided you believe it influenced why you acted in a particular way, it is relevant for this model. Next, write down the consequences of the behaviour. These can be your own actions but also those of others around you.

When you have mapped all these aspects, write down what you could have done to avoid the unpleasant consequences. These might include acting in different ways, both before and after the event, but they can also include thinking about a situation differently, holding yourself and others in a more compassionate light and interpreting evidence in a more considerate way. Everything you note here should mean you will be better prepared to respond, using the interventions you've recorded here, should a similar situation arise in the future.

ABC Analysis for Behavioural Modification

A — Antecedents

- Partner doesn't pick up the phone when I call
- Worried that he might be in danger

Potential interventions on antecedents

- Speak with my partner about why he is unable to answer his phone

B — Behaviours

- Call several times and leave frantic voice messages
- Can't focus on the work I need to do

Potential interventions on behaviours

- Only call once
- Resort to text messages

C — Consequences

- We get into a fight when we both get home

Potential interventions on consequences

- Make sure not to have a conversation about phone etiquette when I am upset

1.10 Problem Development Model

De Shazer, S. (1988). *Clues: Investigating solutions in brief therapy*. New York: Norton & Co.

Purpose

Psychological problems do not come out of nowhere; they have genetic, family, historical, social and environmental roots. It can be useful to identify these factors as this can do much to mitigate the self-critical, self-blaming voice that says, 'It's all my fault' or 'I was born a failure'. If we can recognise the challenges that we faced from birth and in childhood and how they have influenced us down the years, we may be kinder to our adult self and more understanding of our past actions.

It can also be helpful to examine what currently keeps a person vulnerable to psychological problems now. It might be precarious employment, unsuitable accommodation, debt, a toxic or violent relationship, illness or increasing dependency of old age – all these, and other issues, can increase your vulnerability. The purpose of the Problem Development Model is to identify how these might have triggered your problem and how that problem is then maintained either by your actions or by the way you interpret the situation. While there is much in life that is outside our control, our actions and thoughts give us some influence over which direction we take and can sometimes allow us to play the hand that life has dealt us more successfully.

Suitability

The Problem Development Model can be helpful for anyone who wants to focus on the bigger picture and understand how their problems might be affected by their past and current environment. While many maintenance models focus exclusively on the negative aspects of a problem, this model also directs attention towards the protective factors that keep us from spiralling further downwards. This can usefully highlight resources we may not be fully aware of and that we can draw on for additional support.

How to use

Start by writing down your problem. Try to describe it succinctly and in simple terms. If the problem seems too complex to be treated that way, use several copies of the model to address each difficulty separately and make them more manageable. Next, explore the current lifestyle factors that might have made your problem worse. Then ask yourself how those current risks might be influenced by such things as your childhood, your family of origin, your race or culture, your sexuality or gender or perhaps your deep-seated beliefs about the world and yourself.

Once you have got a clearer picture of your circumstances and history, look to focus on the things that are now within your control, that you can do something about, and that are possibly maintaining the problem. This is a crucial step as they most likely will be the focus of future interventions. When this is done, look to the far right of the model and start to list the protective factors in your life that you can call up to keep you grounded and prevent you from slipping into a downward spiral. These can be internal resources, such as character traits and motivation. They can also include family, friends and organisations that have your back and your best interests at heart. It might be that you are not using these protective factors to their full capacity at the moment – give that some thought and consider how you might make more use of them to resolve your problem.

Problem Development Model

What puts me at risk now?

Recently lost my job

Winter affects my mood

Broke up with my partner

What in my life might have made me more vulnerable to this risk?

I have rarely worked in stable jobs

I don't have the best relationship with my family and can't rely on them for support

What is the problem?

I can't motivate myself to get out of bed. I avoid doing the things I need to do

Maintaining factors

I only engage in activities if I'm in the right mood

What are my protective factors?

I have a strong, supportive network of friends

I am physically healthy

I know who to contact if I need help

I have hope for the future

I am a good employee and know that, if I can get a job, I will work hard at it

Formulations 25

1.11 Coping Strategies Model

Folkman, S. (1984). Personal control and stress and coping processes: A theoretical analysis. *Journal of Personality and Social Psychology, 46*(4), 839–852.

Purpose

The purpose of this model is to help you understand why certain problems are maintained. The answer lies in the fact that we often use coping strategies that are unhealthy for us. An unhealthy coping strategy is one that in the long run has consequences that perpetuate and even intensify existing problems. A healthy coping strategy is one that reduces those problems, even if at first it can be unpleasant or difficult to accomplish. To identify which is which, it is necessary to fully understand the consequences of a particular strategy. Then you can make a rational decision either to abandon the strategy or embrace it.

Suitability

We all use coping strategies to resolve our problems. Understanding which coping strategies are healthy and which are unhealthy is an important step towards direct action. I recommend this model as a means to reflect on current coping strategies and their consequences, so as to provide a space where the idea of change can be contemplated.

How to use

Complete one worksheet for each problem. Describe the problem in some detail, and then list what you think are your current unhealthy coping strategies. Many of these might be readily apparent; others may be harder to discern. Coping strategies can be behaviours that you enact, but they can also be reducing or stopping doing something that you would normally do. Doing nothing is a strategy that can serve to remove perceived threats from view and can have significant impact on how you feel, both in the short and long term.

Next, look at your healthy coping strategies. These might be strategies that you are currently using, but they can also include those that you could usefully incorporate into your life. Write down as many as you can think of and imagine what their expected outcomes might be. Hopefully, the outcomes should align with your goals and motivate you to reach out and seize them.

Coping Strategies Model

Current problem

I get very anxious when I am in crowded places like shopping malls and metro stations. I feel the walls are closing in on me and I can't breathe

Unhealthy coping strategies	Consequences of unhealthy coping strategies
Avoid malls and metro stations	I have lost independence. I need to ask others to shop for me. I can't travel around as easily as I did before
I cancel plans with friends	I miss spending time with my friends and feel more lonely
I call my partner if I'm feeling very anxious	I believe this puts a strain on our relationship when I call too often

Potential healthy coping strategies	Expected outcomes of healthy coping strategies
Gradually doing more in certain places	Will feel anxious at first, but hope it will decrease as I get more used to crowds
Practise relaxation exercises	Become more confident in dealing with my anxiety without resorting to outside help
Exercise more outside	Feel more confident and be better able to deal with difficulty breathing

1.12 Biopsychosocial Model of Health

Engel, G. (1977). The need for a new medical model: A challenge for biomedical science. *Science, 196,* 126–129.

Purpose

There is a tendency to think of psychological issues as being entirely in the mind. This is a reductionist philosophy that ignores the complexity of the mind–body inter-relationship. In reality, our motivations, thoughts and self-doubts are informed by the world we live in and our biology. If we ignore this, we risk falling into a trap of believing that we can resolve life's problems simply by thinking positively. Many problems need practical solutions and resources. Similarly, many of our ways of being in the world and dealing with our problems are rooted in our hormones and genetic make-up, and no amount of cognitive restructuring will make them disappear.

Psychological factors do have an important role in maintaining problems. By placing mental health at the centre, the Biopsychosocial Model of Health illustrates the inter-relationship between biological, sociological and psychological factors. It is not a radical idea that our bodies or our upbringings have an influence on how we feel, but sometimes it can take a model such as this to fully reveal the interplay between those factors. And doing so can reduce feelings of blame or disempowerment and allow us to see our issues in a new light.

Suitability

This would be a useful model for people wanting to explore how the psychological intersects with the biological and sociological. If you are using the models in this book alongside medication or receiving some form of social care, this model highlights the holistic nature of support and can help you to think about your problems in new, more multidimensional ways. It is of particular use to people with long-term physical conditions, where their mental health and wellbeing may be influenced by factors outside the strictly psychological. Consider supplementing this model with the material from the Further Support and Resources section at the end of the book.

How to use

As an introduction to understanding mental health, the Biopsychosocial Model of Health can be useful in that it draws attention to the factors that are often neglected in psychological treatment. I suggest you start by listing in each of the main circles your current biological, sociological and psychological problems. This may be harder than you expect, as many of these problems will flow into other circles. If this is the case, use the permeable borders of the circles to list the problems that straddle more than one. Make sure you don't just focus on the visible problems like injury or employment status; include moods, negative thinking patterns and unhealthy coping strategies as well. Consider how one factor might strengthen another, and ask yourself what would happen if you made a change in one circle – what might be the effect on the others?

Formulations 29

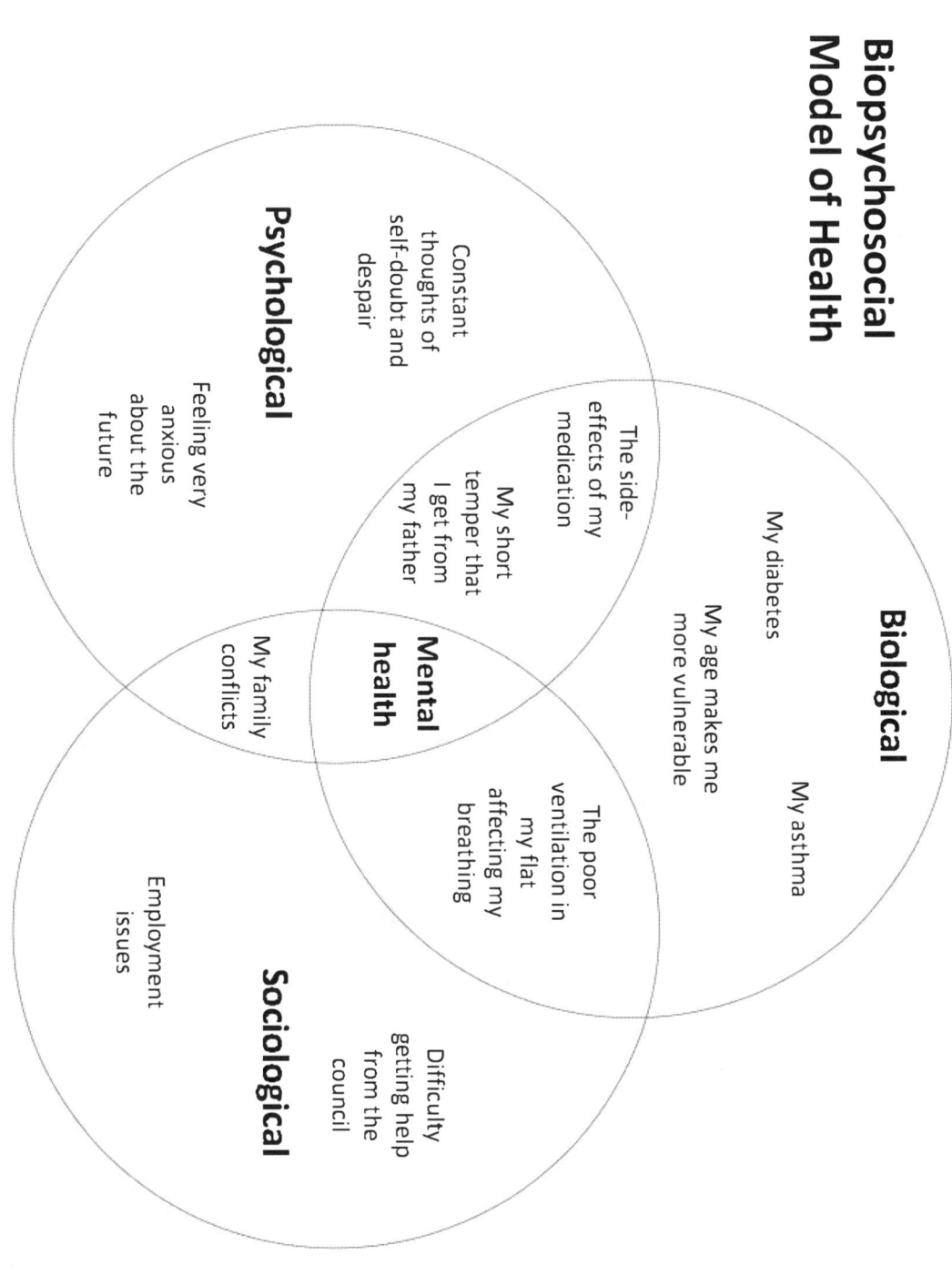

Chapter 2. Goals and behavioural planning

Introduction

Once you have a better understanding of your problems, the question becomes, what now? Being able to name what is troubling you and understand the underlying factors is hugely empowering. After all, knowledge is power. Yet it is only when that knowledge is turned to a purpose that we can truly reap the rewards. This chapter is concerned with transforming knowledge into specific goals. If you are depressed, for instance, knowing this is only beneficial to you if it leads to you taking steps towards recovery. These steps are articulated in the models described in this chapter, not in a prescriptive way – every individual's needs differ – but in a way that encourages you to explore and reflect on what you could do that might help you feel better.

Several of the models described here highlight the need to look at life as a construct made up of distinct parts. Nine Pillars (p.34), for instance, allows you to identify the areas where you are doing well and those where you could do better. Often, we expend all our energy in one direction and neglect other aspects of our life that might be able to provide us with more balance. Reviewing your strengths while becoming conscious of your weaknesses is crucial to being able to prioritise certain activities. If you are finding it particularly difficult to prioritise what is important to you, consider using Stress Quadrant (p.40) to rate them on a scale of urgency and importance, and then using the Behavioural Diary (p.44) to help you schedule them into your day.

Occasionally, recognising what is important can itself be a challenge. When we are suffering, we can easily become disconnected from our values and behave and think in ways that do not reflect who we truly are. Exploring Values (p.50) can act as a helpful reminder of the direction in which we want to take our lives. This can be followed by Value Compass (p.52), which enables us to align our values with specific behaviours that can be practised over the next few weeks. If we can't fulfil our values by our behaviour alone, changing the way we perceive our situation can sometimes be just as helpful. This can be a case of adjusting our expectations of others or what we expect from the world, or being less harsh on ourselves. Reality vs Expectations (p.38) can be useful here for exploring the difference between what we are capable of achieving through action and what requires a change in outlook.

Goal setting can be tough, even when you know the direction you need to go in. Goals can be vague and hard to measure. Sometimes they need to be tied to something concrete so they don't float away. Rephrasing your goals with SMART Goals (p.32) or deciding to focus on a particular aspect of your life such as improving your sleep (Sleep Hygiene Checklist, p.36) can make more challenging goals seem a little more attainable.

At the start, all these changes can seem overwhelming. It can be difficult to know how and where to begin. Suddenly there is a need to be proactive and organise your time better. If you don't already keep a daily schedule, I suggest you do so, as it can be an effective way to track not only what you have been doing but what you want to do in the future. Use a model such as the Behavioural Diary (p.44) to record your progress – but use it honestly! The diary can help increase your motivation and enthusiasm for activities and, combined with Identifying Activities (p.46), can help you explore new activities to engage in that give a sense of pleasure or achievement.

This chapter is designed around the principle that, if you can create a number of specific goals for yourself, you will feel less hopeless and less likely to believe that nothing in your life will ever change. Once you see yourself achieving these goals, your confidence will improve and your sense of autonomy will increase too. Be sure to hold onto the goals you achieve as you progress through the book. It is a powerful feeling to be able to tick off a personal goal, so record any evidence that might sustain that feeling.

2.1 SMART Goals

Locke, E.A. & Latham, G.P. (1994). Goal setting theory. In H.F. O'Neil, Jr. & M. Drillings (Eds.), *Motivation: Theory and research* (pp.13–29). Lawrence Erlbaum Associates.

Purpose

Goals are a great way to increase motivation. If you have a specific aim, you are much less likely to lose enthusiasm for an unpleasant activity if you can tell yourself that it is necessary in order to realise your dream. Unfortunately, goals are often expressed in very abstract terms, and it can be difficult to work out how to approach the larger ones. If your goal is to improve your mental health, for example, you need to break this down into specific steps towards that goal, so you can measure your progress. This will also show you if the goal is relevant and achievable right now.

Setting goals that are too difficult can lead to demoralisation if you don't make the expected progress. It's important to know your limits and adjust your ambitions to your present circumstances. This can be frustrating – when you are feeling low, you just want to snap out of it and return to previous performance levels straight away. Keep this in mind when setting goals and, above all else, be compassionate to yourself if you encounter difficulties when chasing your targets.

Suitability

We all have goals that we want to achieve in life. But if those goals are vague and unspecific, our chances of achieving them diminish. SMART Goals is a practical tool that can help you take your dreams and ambitions and reframe them as specific goals that can be worked towards in the present moment.

How to use

Using one goal per worksheet, work your way from the top to the bottom. As you do so, refine what might start off as a vague dream into something that can be targeted immediately. The following headings should help with that:

- **Specific** – ensure that your goal is specific by using dates, places and resources that you will need to achieve it.

- **Measurable** – make sure that you word your goal in such a way that progress can be measured. If your goal is to feel a certain way, ask yourself what you did in the past when you felt that way. It's much easier to measure behaviours than emotions.

- **Achievable** – ask yourself if your goal is possible to achieve in the short term. If it is a long-term goal, consider breaking it down into smaller steps.

- **Relevant** – check to make sure the goal is relevant to your life now, that it is something that you want to aim towards and that it will make a worthwhile difference to your life.

- **Time specific** – give yourself a deadline to reach the goal. A specific date works best. If this sounds tough, consider revisiting 'specific' and refining your goal further.

SMART Goals

Specific

Exercise at my local gym twice a week, for an hour at a time

Measurable

Keep a record of the times that I attend the gym

Achievable

I have a gym membership. I also have used gyms before and I know what to bring and what to expect

Relevant

I think going to the gym twice a week is a good start to improving how I feel, and once my fitness and motivation improves, I can consider increasing the days per week

Time-limited

I will go to the gym next week. I will reassess this goal in two months' time to see what progress I have made

2.2 Nine Pillars

Byrne, U. (2005). Wheel of life: Effective steps for stress management. *Business Information Review, 22*(2), 123–130.

Purpose

The idea behind Nine Pillars is the metaphor of a temple whose roof is supported by nine pillars. When all nine pillars stand strong, the roof remains supported. If one or two pillars crumble, the roof will begin to crack and fracture. If further pillars collapse, there is a chance that the whole temple will too. Each of these pillars represents an area of your life that promotes wellbeing. It is not necessary to cover every area, but if you notice many that have been neglected, it is worth considering what could be done to change that.

When we are very stressed, we tend to rely increasingly on one or two pillars and expect that they can, on their own, keep the roof supported. Spending all your time at work or expending all your energy on caring for a family member is often necessary, and at times it can be rewarding. But in the long run it can be exhausting, as you have little time to give to yourself. It also makes you vulnerable. If you lose your job or your family member passes away, you have lost not just an important part of your life but also perhaps your reason for getting up in the morning. This can make an already distressing situation feel catastrophic.

The Nine Pillars model can help you identify the areas where you are performing strongly and those where you need to improve. It's important to note that each completed worksheet will look different, as life priorities differ from person to person. There is no ideal balance that ensures good mental health. The purpose of this worksheet is to allow for individual reflection about what is important in your life and to realign those values with what you spend your days doing.

How to use

Begin by writing down the activities you are engaging in at the moment under the relevant headings. You might find that some pursuits belong under more than one heading. Playing football with friends can be classified under exercise, friends or hobbies, for example. Choose the area that you think is most appropriate for it, and do not worry about getting it 'wrong'.

Once you have done this, you may notice that some of the boxes are empty or have less in them than others. If so, use a different coloured pen to write down things that you would like to add to your life in those areas. These might be things that you used to do but have stopped, or activities that you have always wanted to pursue but, for various reasons, have never attempted. Try to be specific and be sure to write down only the activities that are in your power to achieve. This will make it easier to implement the changes going forward.

Suitability

Nine Pillars is helpful if you feel you are leading an imbalanced life where just one or two pillars are supporting all your life. Often you will be expending your energy on other people and neglecting your self-care. This model can help you identify these imbalances and think up ways to correct them. I recommend it as a first step towards dealing with stress; it combines well with SMART Goals (p.32).

Nine Pillars

Contribution	Hobbies	Exercise
I am helping my sister learn how to drive I could volunteer to help out at my local church	I sew I could get back into learning how to play the piano	I practise judo I swim once a week
Family	**Alone time**	**Personal growth**
I visit my family once a week on Sunday for dinner I am helping my sister learn how to drive	I read in the evenings I would like to try meditation to help with my stress	I am taking a course at my local college I am getting further training on how to use the new IT system at work
Work	**Relationship**	**Friends**
I have a good job that I mostly enjoy doing I am getting further training on how to use the new IT system I am thinking about applying for a promotion	N/A I could let my sister arrange a blind date for me	I spend time with my friends at weekends. We see a film or just meet and chat I want to plan a trip to Spain with some close friends

2.3 Sleep Hygiene Checklist

Riedel, B. (2000). Sleep hygiene. In K.L. Lichstein & C.M. Morin (Eds.), *Treatment of late-life insomnia* (pp. 125–146). Sage.

Purpose

A good night's sleep is essential to our physical and mental wellbeing. Too little sleep results in decreased energy, irritability and poor concentration. In fact, there are few things that sleep does not affect. Your body will often respond to stress and anxiety by making it more difficult to fall sleep and stay asleep. This can compound existing problems as you become too tired to deal with them.

There are many reasons why we may struggle to sleep well. One of the most common is our sleep behaviour. Irregular bedtimes, drinking stimulants such as coffee late at night, watching TV, doing any kind of screenwork before sleep and clock-watching in bed can all negatively affect the quality of our sleep. We may have been following these and other bedtime habits for many years, and often it is the accumulation of bad habits topped by a recent stressful life event that stops us sleeping. Too little exercise or an unhealthy diet can also affect our sleep. Often subtle changes in other aspects of our daily life can have a knock-on effect on how much sleep we are able to get.

The Sleep Hygiene Checklist can show us what factors are impacting our sleep and identify behaviours that we might want to change. There is no expectation that every item on the list can be achieved at once, but even if we achieve only a few, it should be taken as a sign that some new habits might be beneficial.

Suitability

One of the most straightforward ways of resolving poor sleep is to change habits and behaviours that might be influencing this. The Sleep Hygiene Checklist can help you identify these and which ones you might be able to change. Even if the problem is anxiety or chronic pain, you may be able to do something towards resolving or managing these. Better sleep may also help you cope better with these difficulties.

How to use

Work your way through the questions, answering 'no', 'somewhat' or 'yes', as relevant. If at the end you notice that most are ticked 'yes', you can regard that as evidence of your healthy sleeping strategies. If many are ticked 'no', then you should ask yourself if these are things that you could change, and if so, how you would go about doing that.

There is space at the end of the checklist to write these reflections down and phrase them as goals. I suggest you choose a few at first and if, in the next few weeks, you are successful in implementing them, you can continue and introduce more. At that point, you should already be seeing a change in how much sleep you are getting. If that is not the case, consider exploring whether stress or anxiety might be the cause of poor sleep. If so, consider using some of the other models in this chapter, such as Stress Quadrant (p.40) or Nine Pillars (p.34) for further support.

Goals and behavioural planning 37

Sleep Hygiene Checkist

Sleep hygiene tips	No	Somewhat	Yes
Regular sleeping timetable	X		
Using the bed only for sleep	X		
Avoiding stimulating activities before sleep		X	
Avoiding caffeine and nicotine before sleep	X		
Avoiding alcohol before sleep			X
No napping during the day			X
Having an evening ritual		X	
Avoiding hot baths before sleep	X		
No clock watching	X		
Using a sleep diary/app		X	
Exercising during the day		X	
Avoiding exercise 4 hours before sleep	X		
Eating a balanced, nutritious diet			X
Making sure the bedroom is dark when sleeping		X	
Making sure to do activities during the day even if tired	X		

Initial sleeping goals

I think a good place to start would be to make sure that I am using my bed just for sleeping and keeping to a strict bedtime. I would like to do more during the day even if I am tired, as sometimes I feel I have too much energy in the evenings. I will also keep my phone away from my bed so I can't check the time/alarm when I have trouble sleeping.

2.4 Reality vs Expectations

Kube, T., Rief, W. & Glombiewski, J.A. (2017). On the maintenance of expectations in major depression: Investigating a neglected phenomenon. *Frontiers in Psychology, 8*(9), doi.org/10.3389/fpsyg.2017.00009

Purpose

It is possible to see all problems in one of two ways. Is this a problem that I can do something about – can I change reality to better suit my needs? Or is this a problem that requires me to change how I look at the world and myself – will changing my expectations result in me feeling better? In practice, mostly a combination of both strategies leads to the best results.

To change your reality, you must first acknowledge the limits to what you can do. Often, we imagine that we can control other people's behaviours by force of personality or persuasion. This can result in failure when the other person (or people) asserts themself and foils our plans. Similarly, we might believe that we can control our emotions by controlling our environment so that nothing unsettling or distressing happens to us. This sets us up for failure as nothing we do can entirely ensure we never experience anything unpleasant – there are too many factors outside our control. So, if you are thinking about how to change your reality, focus on your own behaviours (but not necessarily on the consequences of those behaviours; we can control our actions, but we cannot always foresee their consequences).

If there are things in your reality that you cannot change, your best strategy might be to change your expectations of them. This can involve questioning your assumptions about how dangerous the world really is, or how much responsibility you have for another person's actions. This might seem easier than going out into the world and making changes happen, but it can be very difficult to challenge beliefs that you have held for many years. Thankfully, as this book attests, there are many different ways of going about this.

Suitability

This model helps us establish two clear pathways forward to resolve our problems: change the reality around us or change our expectations of reality. The first encourages proactive decision-making; the second encourages introspection and challenging our beliefs. Both are usually necessary to deal with the issues confronting us. Nevertheless, there is still an art in working out which solution fits best with which problem. Suitable for anyone, Reality vs Expectations is intended to help make those distinctions clearer.

How to use

Reality vs Expectations asks you to look at your life and identify what needs changing and what needs re-evaluating. When it comes to writing down things that need changing, start small. Remember the central tenet: it must be within your control. If obstacles appear that are outside your control, imagine how changing your thinking patterns might reduce the intensity of any negative emotions the obstacles would provoke. For example, if you are always worried that disaster will strike, highlight the catastrophic thinking and your intention to change it. It's fine if you don't have any idea how to do that right now. For the moment, it is enough to recognise what the problem is. When you have finished, you should have a number of improvements and changes written down in each column. The columns might not be the same length; if so, use that as inspiration to guide your next steps. For instance, Thought-Disputing Model (Chapter, 5, p.94) can be useful for managing expectations, while Behavioural Experiment (Chapter 6, p.116) can influence how you see reality and change it too.

Reality vs Expectations

Improve my reality	Change my expectations
Focus on putting myself first for a change	I don't always have to be at 100%
Look after my health better – e.g. exercise three times a week, cook my own meals and eat fewer takeaways	I can't help everyone all the time
Be open and communicative with people close to me	Prioritise what is important and learn to let go and accept what I can't change
Tell my boss that I need to take a holiday	If I disagree with someone, I don't need to feel guilty that I have hurt their feelings
Start allowing my children more independence so they don't rely on me so much	Life is a marathon, not a sprint
Reconnect with friends I have lost touch with	Sometimes people will let me down, but when that happens it is not the end of the world
Work on my time management so that I can find time to do more things with my partner	
Be more assertive when I feel people are taking advantage of me	
Try to keep a regular sleeping pattern	

2.5 Stress Quadrant

Bratterud, H., Burgess, M., Fasy, B.T., Millman, D.L., Oster, T. & Sung, E.C. (2020). The Sung diagram: Revitalizing the Eisenhower matrix. In Pietarinen, A.-V., Chapman, P., Bosveld-de Smet, L., Giardino, V., J Corter, J. & Linker, S. (Eds.), *Diagrammatic representation and inference: 11th International Conference, Diagrams 2020, Tallinn, Estonia, August 24–28, 2020, Proceedings* (pp.498–502). Springer International Publishing.

Purpose

When responsibilities and demands mount up, it can be hard to apply effective time management. If you can't manage your time properly, your stress levels can rise, making you feel overwhelmed and powerless. The Stress Quadrant model is about taking that power back into your hands by reviewing the activities that need to be done and grading them on a four-point scale for urgency and importance. The model demonstrates how to prioritise activities and organise them in such a way that knowing what to do first becomes obvious.

Suitability

Stress Quadrant is very useful for anyone who is under a lot of stress and doesn't know how to manage their responsibilities and time. It is a handy reflective tool that can also be referred back to if new demands arise and threaten to upset your schedule.

How to use

The model is divided into four subsections, listed here in order of priority:

- **Important and urgent** – activities that hold a lot of value for you, but also have a time limit that means they cannot be put off forever. A good example of this would be a work project that has a firm deadline.

- **Important and not urgent** – these activities are important, but they don't have to be done immediately; there will be no repercussions if they are done later instead of now.

- **Not important but urgent** – these are activities that are not crucial to your short- or long-term goals but there is some pressure from others to complete them soon. They may be demands placed on you by others, or appointments that you think you can miss without regret or repercussions.

- **Not important and not urgent** – often trivial things that can be done sometime in the future and if you don't do them, you won't regret it, so they can most likely be further postponed.

Begin by listing the important and urgent activities, then work your way through the rest of the worksheet until you have written down all your current obligations. Now identity those activities with the highest priority, those that are less urgent, and so on, completing all four quadrants. This is the most systematic way of completing the worksheet, but ultimately you have the freedom to pick and choose what you do first. Use the model as a guide, not a taskmaster that adds to your stress.

Stress Quadrant

Important and urgent

Finish my essay by the deadline

Look for a new flatmate so we don't have an empty room in our flat

Reply to the recent job offer I was given

Important and not urgent

Get a first for my degree

Ask for advice from the university careers service

Book my annual sight check with the optician

Not important and urgent

Help a classmate with handing in their assignment

Make sure I don't miss my favourite TV show

Get to lectures early so I can sit near the front

Let my friend know if I can come to their party

Not important and not urgent

Get a haircut

Buy some new shoes

2.6 Phobia Ladder

Kircanski, K., Mortazavi, A., Castriotta, N., Baker, A.S., Mystkowski, J.L., Yi, R. & Craske, M.G. (2012). Challenges to the traditional exposure paradigm: Variability in exposure therapy for contamination fears. *Journal of Behavior Therapy and Experimental Psychiatry, 43*(2), 745–751.

Purpose

A phobia is a pronounced and recurring fear of an object, place, situation or creature. It is characterised by an unrealistic appraisal of the dangers that the object, place, situation or creature presents. In this way it is different from fear, which is an emotion we feel when confronted with a very real and imminent danger. For example, if you were confronted by a dog that was visibly aggressive and wasn't on a lead or in anyone's control, a certain amount of fear would generally be regarded as a rational response, as would certain coping strategies, such as running away. But if you are afraid of all dogs, no matter what the situation is – one dog or many dogs, large dogs or small ones, whether the dog is awake and growling or fast asleep – this would mostly likely be seen as a phobia. Running away from a small, sleeping dog would be regarded as a phobic reaction, with no rational basis.

Phobias can devastate a person's life. They can keep us housebound and in a state of perpetual terror. Fortunately, they can be overcome. One of the best strategies for doing this is called graded exposure – briefly, listing your fears in a line from least to greatest and then exposing yourself to those fears in that order. You begin with the fears that are the most manageable and, by overcoming them, you build up the confidence to tackle the more difficult ones. Phobia Ladder is a helpful guide to this process of listing these fears and assigning them a rating, thereby laying the foundations for all future graded exposure exercises.

Suitability

Phobia Ladder is a great introduction to graded exposure as it ranks your fears on a spectrum, with the worst fears at the top of the ladder and the most manageable at the bottom. The model works best with phobias, as less systematic fears are not so easily separated out and categorised. When you have completed the model, you can combine it with the Graded Exposure for Phobias worksheet in Chapter 6 (p.130).

How to use

Make a list of all the scenarios that your fear prevents you from engaging in. If you have claustrophobia, for example, imagine all the environments in which you experience severe anxiety or that you avoid at all costs. Pick a scenario that causes significant fear and rank that fear on a scale of 0 to 100. If you give it, say, 70, put it at the top of the medium-feared section; 30 would be around the middle of the least feared section.

Next, imagine a scenario that would cause you greater fear or less fear. It might be the same scenario with a friend by your side, or it might be the same scenario at night. In either instance, the change might inch the fear rating up or down a few degrees. You might also want to list another scenario that is entirely different from the first. As long as the underlying fear remains the same, that is all that matters. Keep progressing in this manner until you have filled up the entire model with feared scenarios and given each a rating.

The model deliberately excludes anything that you would rate at less than 20, as such a low score might not make a scenario fearful enough to warrant exposure to it. When completing the model, be sure to include a balance of scenarios across all three difficulty levels. If the scenarios all have a high difficulty rating, you might find it hard to make the first few steps. When you have completed the model, it should be quite clear which scenarios you should start exposing yourself to first. At this point you could begin using the Graded Exposure for Phobias worksheet in Chapter 6 (p.130)

Phobia Ladder

Fear rating	Activity hierarchy	0-100
Most feared – 75-100	Going to a packed concert; standing in the front row	100
	Being in a lift packed with people	100
	Being in an empty lift	90
	Being on a crowded train	80
	Being on a crowded bus	80
Medium feared – 50-75	Being in a crowd on the street	70
	Walking in the park with a lot of joggers and cyclists going past	65
	Being in a supermarket queue	65
	Being in a locked car	55
	Being in a locked room, e.g. bathroom	50
Least feared – 20-50	Being at a friend's crowded party	40
	Being in my living room with a lot of guests	35
	Being in a small room without windows	25
	Having all the windows and doors closed when I am trying to sleep	25
	Being at the centre of a conversation in a group	20

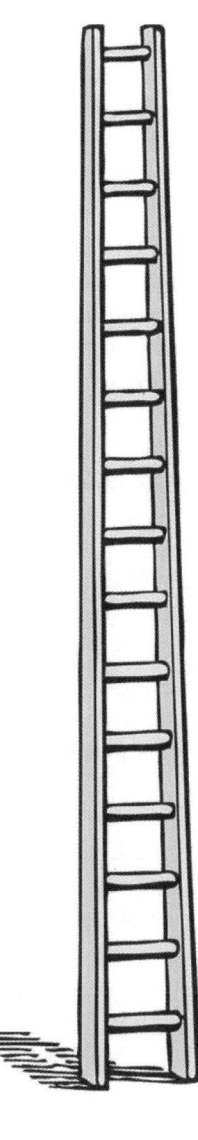

2.7 Behavioural Diary

Lejuez, C.W., Hopko, D.R. & Hopko, S.D. (2001). A brief behavioral activation treatment for depression: Treatment manual. *Behavior Modification, 25*(2), 255–286.

Purpose

When we feel low, we tend to isolate ourselves and stop doing things. We feel too tired or can't be bothered. We cancel social plans and neglect responsibilities because we can't see the point. While this might provide some temporary relief, we may find we have abandoned the activities that gave us a sense of pleasure or accomplishment, and this in itself can lead to depression, as our mood spirals downwards. To put things right, we have to identify the helpful activities we have stopped and restart them. Doing this can highlight the link between our behaviour and our mood. When you see how your mood is linked to what you do, it can motivate you to change your behaviour to improve your mood.

Suitability

Keeping a record of what you do during the week can be a useful reflection tool. Similarly, most people can see the benefit of planning activities in advance, and more so if they know they are likely to avoid them otherwise. In general, the Behavioural Diary works best for people who have low motivation, lack a routine and tend to procrastinate. It can be an effective introduction to recognising the role that behaviour plays in reinforcing depression.

How to use

The Behavioural Diary can be used in one of two ways: to review what you do during the day, and to plan your upcoming week:

1) Review of the day

At the end of each day, record what you have done. Dividing the morning, afternoon and evening into two slots each stops the diary from becoming too detailed. Similarly, the prompts 'what', 'where' and 'who' encourage you to focus on the essence of what you were doing. In each slot, you can score the activity on a scale of 1–10, to rate how you felt when doing the activity (1 = very distressing; 10 = tremendously enjoyable). Do this every day for a week, then look back and see if any patterns or insights emerge.

2) Plan your week

At the start of the week, write down everything that you would like to do in the coming seven days. This can be a mix of routine, pleasurable and necessary activities. Try to ensure you have an even balance of difficult, moderate and easy across the week. If you are planning some quite difficult activities, offset their difficulty with more easily accomplished activities on either side. Then put the diary where you can see it or take a photo of it on your phone. As you start the week, try to follow what's in the diary as much as possible. You might find your enthusiasm for some tasks is quite low. That's fine. If that is the case, tell yourself to follow your plan, not your mood, and attempt the task anyway. Often the biggest challenge is starting a task; keeping going is a little easier.

Behavioural Diary

	Monday	Tuesday	Wednesday	Thursday	Friday	Saturday	Sunday
Morning **What:** **Where:** **Who:**	Breakfast, shower, get ready for work 5	Wake up early for morning jog, alone 6	Breakfast, shower, get ready for work 5	Cycle to work, alone 7	Breakfast, shower, get ready for work 6	Sleep in 7	Take family to museum 5
Morning **What:** **Where:** **Who:**	Work 6	Work 6	Work 4	Work 6	Work 5	Go for jog with partner 9	Take family to museum 7
Afternoon **What:** **Where:** **Who:**	Work 6	Work 6	Work 5	Work 6	Work 5	Go for weekend shop 7	Take family to museum 7
Afternoon **What:** **Where:** **Who:**	Work 6	Work 7	Work 4	Work 6	Work 6	Do weekend chores around the house 6	Go through financial records 4
Evening **What:** **Where:** **Who:**	Help children with their homework at home 7	Make dinner with family 8	Pick up children from after-school activities 7	Watch movie with family 8	Go drinking with work colleagues 8	Get babysitter, take partner to restaurant 7	Get takeaway with family 6
Evening **What:** **Where:** **Who:**	Read a book, alone 6	Watch some TV with partner 8	Talk to parents on the phone 6	Read a book, alone 7	Go drinking with work colleagues 8	At home, talk with my partner about their week 7	Have an early night 6

2.8 Identifying Activities

Beck, A.T. (1979). *Cognitive therapy of depression*. Guilford Press.

Purpose

Identifying Activities is designed to help you reintroduce activities into your life. Often when we feel depressed, we stop activities and isolate ourselves from others. This can make us more depressed, and the longer it continues, the harder it is to reverse the process and restart activities we once enjoyed. Activities that we would once have done without thought can become arduous and exhausting, making it even harder for us to do them. The solution is to identify the activities we have stopped, categorise them according to their role in our life, and then grade them in terms of difficulty. This can make the seemingly impossible look possible and within reach. When using this worksheet, it is important to set yourself reasonable expectations and be compassionate with the results. It can be frustrating to discover that previously simple tasks are now so much harder to complete. But, with time and effort, progress can be made.

Suitability

This worksheet is ideal for people who have decided to increase the range and challenge of their daily behaviours. Identifying Activities provides a systematic approach to behavioural modification. I recommend using this worksheet alongside the Behavioural Diary (p.44). First you identify what you would like to do and assess the difficulty, and then you plan your coming week in the diary.

How to use

The worksheet is divided into two sections. The first consists of three types of activities: routine, pleasurable and necessary. A routine activity is something that you do frequently, perhaps every day, and usually involves little thought (e.g. laundry, showering, shaving and so forth). A pleasurable activity is something that you do for fun or to relax, whether alone or with others. Necessary activities are obligations to yourself or others that, if you don't do them, will have adverse effects (e.g. going to work or paying your bills). This division is somewhat arbitrary, but it highlights the need for balance when reintroducing behaviours. For instance, if you don't do anything for pleasure, you might find other activities do not lift your mood and so become something to be endured.

Once you have listed a number of routine, pleasurable and necessary activities, decide which would be the easiest to do and which would be the hardest. When energy and motivation are low, we sometimes try to jumpstart the body and mind by attempting to return to our normal habits. Yet, much like a sprinter with a broken ankle, the road to recovery has to be a gradual process. We wouldn't expect the sprinter to be back on the track after a week in bed. The same goes for when we are trying to recover from depression. It is far better to gradually reintroduce more manageable activities into our schedule. If we try to do everything at once and expect our mood to lift immediately, and then fail, we will end up in a worse place.

Goals and behavioural planning 47

Identifying Activities

Routine	Pleasurable	Necessary
Shower	Play football	Pay the bills
Go shopping for food	Play board games	Fix up things around the house
Cook	Go to the gym	Pick up parents from the airport
Get properly dressed in the morning	Read a magazine	Make appointment with GP
Do laundry	Spend time with friends at local café	Take children to school
Water the plants	Get in touch with old friend over the phone	Call work to let them know I am ill
Do the recycling	Play the guitar	
	Take the dog for a walk	

⬇

Easiest	Medium	Hardest
Shower	Go shopping for food	Play football
Get properly dressed in the morning	Cook	Spend time with friends at local café
Do laundry	Do the recycling	Fix up things around the house
Water the plants	Play board games	Take children to school
Read a magazine	Go to the gym	
Play the guitar	Get in touch with old friend over the phone	
Make appointment with GP	Take the dog for a walk	
Call work to let them know I am ill	Pay the bills	
	Pick up parents from the airport	

2.9 Alternative Solutions Model

Nezu, A.M., Nezu, C.M. & D'Zurilla, T.J. (2013). *Problem-solving therapy: A treatment manual.* Springer.

Purpose

Faced with a difficult problem, we can become paralysed by indecision. It can seem as if there is no easy choice to be made; that any choice will result in negative consequences. But if we do nothing, the issue will drag on forever. In these situations, you have to weigh up the strengths and weaknesses of each solution and decide, as objectively as possible, on a course to take. Every choice will have strengths and weaknesses, but it should be possible to see that some weaknesses are more significant than others and should be avoided at all costs, and some strengths are aligned more closely with your values and goals and so should be favoured over others.

Alternative Solutions Model is designed to help with the practical task of making difficult choices. However, it will only work with problems that are within your control and can be influenced by your choices. Good examples would be changing jobs, leaving the parental home and ending an unhappy relationship. Poor examples would be changing others' behaviours or beliefs and trying to stop yourself feeling specific emotional responses. The model can be used both with simple problems that only have a few clear choices and with complex problems where the weighing of strengths and weaknesses might not readily provide an answer.

Suitability

This model is suitable for anyone who is anxious and facing difficulties that do not have one clear answer. It can help make life choices easier to grasp by providing an opportunity to weigh up each possible choice or solution by what it might cost and what you might gain from it.

How to use

Start by selecting a problem. Be sure to make it as specific as possible. If you feel that this does not fully describe the nature of the problem, use further copies of the worksheet to capture other aspects of it. Once you have your problem written down, list as many solutions to it as you can. Don't censor yourself – if ridiculous ideas come to mind, write them down. When you come to comparing and contrasting them with other solutions, they can make your choice seem clearer.

Once you have a number of solutions, work through them, listing their strengths and weaknesses. These might be practical issues, such as lack of funds. Or they could be matters of personal preference. Both are valid, but how much emphasis you give to each is up to you. After a while it should become clear that there are only a few options really open to you. Consider now how important to you each of the strengths and weaknesses of each solution are. There is no straightforward formula for this calculation, but it can help to imagine a future version of yourself that has accomplished everything that you want in life. Ask yourself, what would that version of me have done to get where they are now? Which choice would they have made here? Use that insight to decide how to move forward and resolve the problem.

Alternative Solutions Model

Specific problem:	I need to find a new place to live		

Possible solution	Strengths	Weaknesses	Yes/no
Contact the council and be put on a waiting list for a property	Council accommodation would be within my budget Relatively simple to check my suitability	Might be a very long wait before they find me a suitable place A lot of bureaucracy and paperwork	No
Move back with my family	I could negotiate a reasonable rent It would be good to spend more time with my younger siblings	I would lose a lot of independence I would feel like I had failed	No
Rent privately	I could quickly find a place that would suit my needs	I would have to reduce my expenses drastically I would not be able to afford anywhere spacious	Yes
Rent privately outside London	More choice of property that is within my budget	I would lose contact with my friends and family I would lose access to the job market in London	No
Get a mortgage on a property	I would have my own place and could decorate it however I liked	I don't have enough for a deposit It's something I always imagined doing jointly with a partner	No

2.10 Exploring Values

Wilson, K.G. & Murrell, A.R. (2004). Values work in acceptance and commitment therapy: Setting a course for behavioral treatment. In S.C. Hayes, V.M. Follette & M. Linehan (Eds.), *Mindfulness and acceptance: Expanding the cognitive-behavioral tradition* (pp.120–151). Guilford Press.

Purpose

A value is a fundamental belief that guides us through life. Our values are embedded in our idea of who we are as person and, unlike opinions or intrusive thoughts, they are quite resistant to change. Regardless, our values do not come to us fully formed; they are created by our environment, character and intentions. Since our values can come from such diverse sources, at times they do not always align with each other, and this can cause a great deal of tension. If you have been taught that what society values is ambition and opportunism, but your mother's values of reserve and humility tell you the opposite, it can be hard to know which direction to take.

The Exploring Values model will help you review the varied values that have influenced your life. By following its path, you can better see what has influenced your own values. This can result in a deeper understanding of yourself and your inner conflicts. It can also point to any interpersonal issues and reveal where change is needed. Ultimately, the model allows you to see yourself from another perspective, and that is always illuminating.

Suitability

This model allows you to explore your values and understand the history behind them. If you are able to see your values as something organic that develops with time, it is easier to imagine how other aspects of your life might be susceptible to change too.

How to use

Begin by exploring the values of your parents or primary caregiver(s). These people often have a significant influence on your own values in the sense that you adopt what they hold to be important, or you resist and make your own path in opposition. Either approach makes listing what they believe(d) crucial to understanding yourself.

Next explore the values of someone you respect. This can be someone you know, or it can be someone whose reputation you are aware of and admire. We often model ourselves on others, especially in our adolescence, and that influence can have a lasting effect. After you have listed a few values there, move on and reflect on the values of your society/culture. These values might be hard to identify unless you live outside your own culture or travel frequently, as it is only when we see ourselves reflected in the eyes of others that our own values tend to spring into relief.

For the final two sections, focus on drawing out any incongruity between the values you live by and those that you aspire to. Some people may manage to live in perfect harmony with their values and never violate them, but most of us fail constantly to live up to our own standards. This is understandable and only human. Nevertheless, discovering how and where we fall short can help us understand our current emotional state better.

Exploring Values

My mother's values

To be caring to others

To always look your best no matter how you feel

Family is everything

The values of someone I respect

You have to put your own desires to one side to be truly great

The ends sometimes justify the means

My father's values

If you work hard, you will achieve success

Every problem can be solved

Never complain

Societal/cultural values

You don't discuss problems with those outside the family

We are judged on our performance, not who we are

The values that I live by

I should always give 100%

Weakness is unacceptable

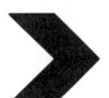

The values I aspire to live by

To be more accepting of my emotions

To be open and honest with others

2.11 The Value Compass

Wilson, K.G. & Murrell, A.R. (2004). Values work in acceptance and commitment therapy: Setting a course for behavioral treatment. In S.C. Hayes, V.M. Follette & M. Linehan (Eds.), *Mindfulness and acceptance: Expanding the cognitive-behavioral tradition* (pp.120–151). Guilford Press.

Purpose

A compass is a tool that guides you in the direction you wish to go. This model does something similar. Instead of relying on the earth's magnetic field, though, it relies on your values to direct your behaviours. A value is a strong, aspirational belief that we use to guide the important decisions in our life. It is not something that always filters through to consciousness, and because of this we can easily engage in activities and behaviours that do not align with our values. The purpose of this model is to remind you of your values and help you identify the behaviours that are true to them and those that go astray.

When contemplating what a value is, it can be helpful to contrast it with strengths. Imagine that you are celebrating your 80th birthday with friends and family. One after another, they stand up and give a speech in your praise. What would you like them to say about you? You may pride yourself on being reliable and organised, for instance, and see these as strengths. Nevertheless, after a long life, we probably would not want to be remembered for these alone. Values should be ideals that we would be proud to think our life represents and would want our friends and family to celebrate and remember us by.

Suitability

When we feel directionless in life, it can be useful to turn our attention to our values. Once we understand that our actions lead us either towards our values or further away from them, we can make changes that form the first tentative steps towards realising who we are and who we wish to be. This model can be paired with Exploring Values (p.50) to learn more about our deepest-seated beliefs.

How to use

First choose one of your values that you wish to focus on. For example:

- caring
- freedom
- loyalty
- connection
- creativity
- courage
- compassion
- fitness
- professionalism
- love
- wisdom
- patience
- flexibility
- autonomy
- wellness
- gratitude
- grace
- honesty
- open-mindedness
- kindness
- collaboration
- ambition
- communication
- learning

Use one of the above, or another value that you hold dear, and write it down on the worksheet. Now ask yourself what actions you can take that will get you closer to realising that value. Keep in mind that a value is not something you will ever possess or embody. It is something that you can hold, like a compass, to direct your activities and lifestyle. While some activities might move you towards your values, others might have the opposite effect. This is why it is important to write down the counterproductive activities on the worksheet too. Perhaps you recognise some of them as ways you are currently behaving. If that is the case, consider reducing or stopping those behaviours so you can move closer towards your value.

I suggest you complete a few Value Compass worksheets, as you may then spot certain behaviours that feature in more than one. These should be highlighted for change, as changing them will be the quickest way of making progress in your life.

Goals and behavioural planning 53

Value Compass

Name of value: Compassion

Towards your value...

Volunteer at my local homeless shelter

Really listen to my partner when they are sharing their day with me

Not be so quick to judge others when they say something I don't agree with

Away from your value...

Isolate myself from others — e.g. avoid the work Christmas party

Ignore the homeless on my commute

Talk over other people in conversation with them

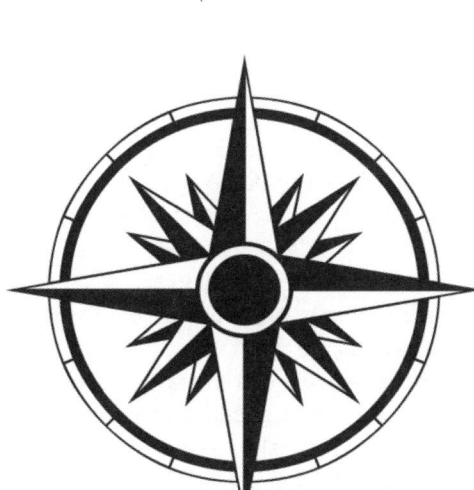

Chapter 3. Relaxation

Introduction

When you make the decision to confront your problems, you are abandoning the avoidance strategies that protected you from anxiety or discomfort and leaving yourself exposed to your fears. This is a very difficult thing to do. When you reflect on what is at the root of your problems and set yourself goals to accomplish, you are challenging your previous coping strategies and opening yourself up to the uncertainty that comes with trying something new. It is essential that you have some basic tools to help you manage how you feel in those moments. This chapter suggests some relaxation strategies that you can use to reduce the intensity of strong emotional reactions.

The exercises in this chapter focus on redirecting your attention away from your thoughts. This immediately indicates when and where relaxation strategies should be applied. If you are being chased by a bear through a forest, the threat to your life is very much present and real. Pausing to breathe and centre yourself will allow the bear to catch up with you. As you are dealing with an actual threat, running as fast as you can should be your first course of action. If, on the other hand, you are anxiously thinking about an upcoming medical appointment and what the outcome might be, the threat is perceived and not actual, and there is little that you can do to resolve the issue. Despite the differences in these threats, your body will respond in a very similar way. The fight/flight response will kick in and you will become hypervigilant to any and all possible threats to your safety. It is in such latter situations that you need to redirect your attention away from your thoughts. Fortunately, there are several simple methods that can help.

Some of the best-known relaxation strategies involve regulating your breathing. When you are anxious, your breathing can get faster and shallower – your lungs are telling you that you need to get more oxygen into your system to prepare you for danger. If you are able to take your attention away from your negative thoughts and towards controlling your breathing, you will quickly see a difference in how you feel. Square Breathing Technique (p.56) and Body Scan (p.62) emphasise the relationship between conscious breathing and mood management.

While focusing on breathing might work well for some people, occasionally it can lead to frustration as results are slow to appear. In these cases, consider taking your attention to your muscles. Just like your breathing, your muscles too are affected by the fight/flight response. They will often tense up and remain so for long periods of time, causing aches and pains, and even headaches. Use Progressive Muscle Relaxation (p.60) to focus on releasing the tension in your muscles and to take your attention away from any worries or rumination.

These methods all involve turning your focus away from your thoughts and towards your body, but in some cases your stress might be coming from an excessive focus on your health. In this situation, consider using relaxation strategies that direct your attention outwards, away from yourself and either towards your surroundings or to activities that you can easily engage in. Mundane Task Focusing (p.64) and Grounding (p.66) both offer means to incorporate outward focus in your daily life.

There is a misconception that relaxation strategies are themselves an avoidance strategy and that they don't, in fact, solve anything. This is a legitimate concern as, when you stop using these strategies, often your negative thoughts will return, and it will seem that you are back where you started. The relaxation strategies in this chapter are not meant as long-term solutions to your problems; rather, they are a way to reinforce the idea that you have some control over how and when you feel upset. Once you have recognised your ability to manage your thoughts, you can approach later chapters in this book with more confidence in your ability to stay calm.

3.1 Square Breathing Technique

Jha, R.K., Acharya, A. & Nepal, O. (2018). Autonomic influence on heart rate for deep breathing and valsalva maneuver in healthy subjects. *Journal of the Nepal Medical Association, 56*(211), 670–673.

Purpose

When anxious or stressed, our bodies activate what is called the fight/flight response. This is an automatic physiological reaction that is designed to keep us safe from threats. Unfortunately, it can be triggered by imagined threats as well as actual ones, and once it begins, it can take some time for the body to return to normal. When your body is in this state, you may experience a rush of adrenaline, your muscles may tense up, your heart beat faster and your digestive system close down. These can all be very alarming and unpleasant.

One of the most common responses is a change in our breathing. We begin to take shorter, faster breaths as our lungs seeks to pump more oxygen into our blood to prepare us for flight or fight. The only problem is that most modern dilemmas cannot be resolved by running away or physical combat. When we are worried about the distant future, for instance, there is usually no way that we can tackle the problem in the present. Similarly, if we have been summoned to see our manager about a workplace problem, running away won't help in the long term and fighting certainly won't help at all; we need to stay calm in order to present our perspective coherently. But we are stuck with all the adrenaline flowing through our system and no way to release it through decisive action. All we can do is redirect our attention elsewhere.

One of the simplest ways of redirecting our attention away from perceived threats is to focus on our breathing. By focusing on slowing down our breathing, we can reverse the fight/flight response, as we are no longer paying attention to whatever caused the initial anxiety. When our breathing slows, we usually start to see any other unpleasant symptoms fade into the background. This will produce the comforting thought that everything is getting back to normal and that we will be fine. Where our body leads, our mind will follow.

Suitability

This breathing technique can be used by anyone to quickly centre themselves and restore their equilibrium. If you are prone to anxiety, you will find the technique helpful in most situations where you need to slow your breathing. Similarly, if you are experiencing panic attacks, you can use it to turn your attention towards your breath and away from any perceived threats. The technique can become a regular part of your routine, or you can use it in a crisis. Fundamentally, its greatest strength is its versatility and wide-ranging applicability.

How to use

Square Breathing Technique can be used in any situation that might cause distress. I suggest you practise it when you are in a positive mood, so that you will be confident you can use the technique correctly when you are feeling anxious or stressed. There is space on the worksheet to add your reflections on this practice.

Start by taking a deep breath in through your nose. Aim for a 3–4-second inhalation. Focus on fully engaging your stomach and abdominal muscles, so that your breath is gathered from your diaphragm and fills your lungs more effectively. Hold that breath for another 3–4 seconds, not letting it go or breathing in further. Exhale from your mouth, again for 3–4 seconds, and then focus on the stillness around you. Repeat as many times as necessary until whatever caused your anxiety feels less intense. Remember, breathing does not solve your problems, but by countering the fight/flight response, it can make you more able to manage your problems.

Square Breathing Technique

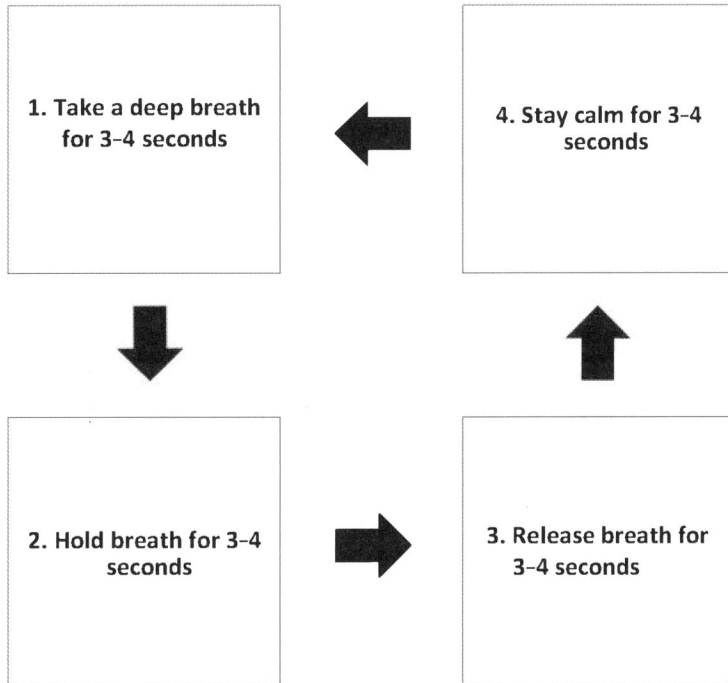

Reflections

I decided to use the square breathing technique when I was on public transport, as that is when my anxiety is at its highest. I found that, when I was focusing on my breathing, I wasn't looking around as much at how crowded the bus was getting. I tried breathing in through my nose and out through my mouth, like I was taught at yoga. My anxiety decreased, but my mind would wander and I would have to snap it back to my breathing. I said to myself 'Stay calm' and that internal reminder helped slow my breathing down. I've noticed in the past that when I get anxious my heart rate and breathing rise together, and when I slow my breathing, my heart rate stays more regular, which makes me feel more in control of what is going on.

3.2 Visual Imagery

Ronen, T. (2011). *The positive power of imagery: Harnessing client imagination in CBT and related therapies.* Wiley-Blackwell.

Purpose

When we are seized by strong emotions, we can feel overwhelmed and hopeless. To make the emotions go away, we often resort to short-term strategies that make things worse. It is worth exploring alternative coping devices, such as relaxation exercises, which can provide you with more effective long-term ways to manage these strong emotions.

Visual Imagery is an exercise that redirects focus from your source of stress towards an interior image: a place where you feel peace. Negative emotions gain strength from our thoughts. If we feel low, we start to judge ourselves and question our value. These thoughts feed the fire. To extinguish a fire, you need to deprive it of fuel. By focusing your attention on a specific mental image, you put a stop to those self-critical thoughts, and this in turn reduces the intensity of the emotions and eventually puts out the fire.

The mind is only capable of focusing on one or two things at a time. Ultimately, it is much better if it focuses on a positive mental image than on the source of the stress. This way of responding does not come naturally; your mind may need a bit of training and practice. With time, though, you will find yourself more and more capable of applying selective attention in moments of distress.

Suitability

Visual Imagery can be used when you are thinking of the future and imagining worst-case scenarios. It can also be used to counter rumination about the past. People who are experiencing constant low-level anxiety may find this exercise can interrupt their maintenance cycles and put them in a better headspace.

How to use

Start this worksheet when you are feeling relatively well. Ensure that you are somewhere that you feel comfortable and allow yourself to close your eyes. Choose a place in your mind that gives you a sense of peace. This can be a place and time in your past or somewhere you imagine yourself in the future, or it can be an entirely fictional location. The only thing that is essential is that you do not associate the place with anxiety or stress or any other negative emotions.

Now you have that place in mind, imagine yourself getting to it. Does it involve a walk across a beach? Does it involve a car journey down a long, winding road? Try to layer the images with as much detail as you can. Eventually you reach your chosen place. Picture what it feels like to step over the threshold. What do your senses pick up? If it is a building with many rooms, wander through each and absorb the atmosphere. Pay attention to how you feel throughout this process. After you notice a feeling of contentedness, make the active decision to withdraw, taking the same route back that brought you there.

Open your eyes. Check your body. Ask yourself how you feel. Are there any changes? Once you have practised this exercise, try it whenever you feel overwhelmed. You do not have to close your eyes if you don't feel it's necessary. You might also find that the more you practise, the less time you have to spend in your safe place before you feel better. This is a positive sign that you are getting better at disentangling yourself from critical thoughts and the strong emotions that often follow.

Visual Imagery

Begin by deciding on a private place in your mind that gives you peace

Imagine the journey to get to that place

Enter your private place

Imagine the return home

Reflections

I decided to try the visual imagery during my lunch breaks, when I knew I would have some time to sit outside alone. I felt a little silly closing my eyes, so I kept them open and focused on a holiday that I had gone on when I was feeling less stressed. Once I had that place in mind, I imagined the flight, the car journey to the resort, even walking up to the villa and opening the front door. I tried to explore all the rooms, and as I did so memories resurfaced around how happy I had been there. It made me a little sad, as the contrast to how I felt now was strong. I made an effort, though, to return to how I had felt there and the feeling of security and wonder that had filled me. I then imagined returning and coming back to my life here. Though I felt a little regretful at what I was giving up, I took those positive feelings I felt at the villa and brought them back to the present. When I stopped doing the imagery work, I felt less stressed and more confident to face the day.

3.3 Progressive Muscle Relaxation

Bernstein, D.A. & Borkovec, T.D. (1973). *Progressive relaxation training: A manual for the helping professions*. Research Press.

Purpose

When the fight/flight response is activated, our muscles prepare for action. There is increased blood flow around the body, and much of that blood is allocated to the larger muscles in preparation for either running away or fighting. Occasionally our muscles might start to spasm, but if they don't, this process remains largely unconscious. Our attention will generally be on whatever triggered the fight/flight response in the first place or trying to understand the significance of the threat, and we will be lost in our worries and critical thinking. Meanwhile, our muscles become more and more tense. This can lead to pain and discomfort, not just in the moment but later on in the day when we are feeling less stressed.

A solution to this pain and to the initial anxious response is Progressive Muscle Relaxation. The technique should be used when the anxiety is at its peak and it involves, like all relaxation strategies, a redirecting of attention towards something other than the perceived threat or worry: in this case, towards your muscles. By focusing on tensing and releasing your muscles in time with your breathing, you become more centred in the present and less focused on any perceived threat. It might seem contrary to common sense to tense your muscles in order to become more relaxed. Yet, by bringing this involuntary process to consciousness, you can quite quickly feel the difference between a tense and relaxed state, and can change one for the other more easily.

Suitability

Progressive Muscle Relaxation will be of benefit to anyone who needs to improve their ability to manage stress and anxiety. It can also help reduce the after-effects of stress or anxiety, such as muscle tension or cramps later in the day.

How to use

Begin by choosing a specific muscle. If there is one that seems to get noticeably tense when your anxiety levels are high, choose that one. Alternatively, start with your calf muscles and, as the exercise progresses, work your way up your body. You can do this technique standing, but it can be easier to practise while sitting.

Flex and stretch the selected muscle, allowing it to relax. Then tense it and hold that tension for at least three to five seconds. As you do this, breathe in for the same amount of time. Release the tensed muscle and exhale for another 3–5 seconds. Note any change in how you feel. Then move on to another muscle. Repeat the same sequence. You can go through most of your body this way, making sure to focus your attention on your muscles and your breathing. The muscles in your face especially are worth tensing and relaxing, as we often carry a lot of stress there.

Once you have finished the entire sequence, which can take up to 20 minutes, depending on your routine, ask yourself how you feel. Hopefully any anxiety that you were previously feeling has diminished. Make a mental note of any success and try to recall this exercise the next time you feel overwhelmed.

Progressive Muscle Relaxation

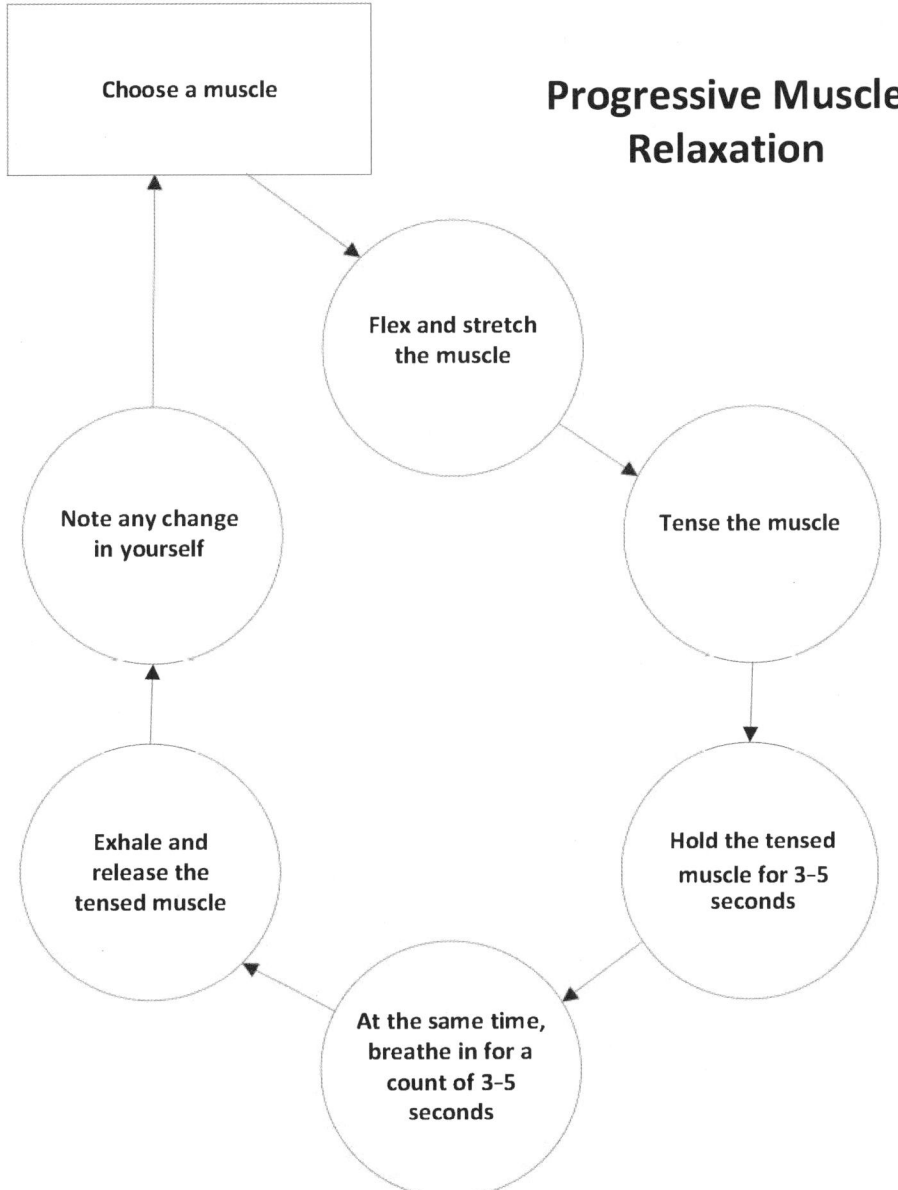

Reflections

When doing the muscle relaxation, it became very apparent how much tension I was carrying in my shoulders and upper back. I sit down for most of the day, in front of a computer, and I think my body starts to cave in and hunch over as the day progresses. This might be why I feel so irritable and on edge in the evenings. When I released each muscle, I tried to picture the source of tension and stress seeping out of the muscle and floating off into the distance. This helped me feel more restored and less anxious and served as a reminder that I need to set more time aside for self-care.

3.4 Body Scan

Kabat-Zinn, J. & Hanh, T.N. (2009). *Full catastrophe living: Using the wisdom of your body and mind to face stress, pain, and illness.* Random House Publishing Group.

Purpose

Our bodies are depositories for stress. When we are working very hard, balancing countless obligations and spending our days over-analysing problems, our bodies bear the brunt of our labours. When we feel overwhelmed, our bodies will communicate this to us in certain ways. We might find it hard to sleep, experience painful headaches or lose interest in activities and struggle to concentrate. Instead of heeding our bodies, we often ignore these symptoms and carry on regardless. This can result in the symptoms becoming worse, not better.

When crisis strikes, the solution is to refocus your attention not on your problems but on your neglected body. Body Scan can be used when you are feeling at your worst. It works by encouraging you to listen to your body and scan it for signs of tension and discomfort. This is done through controlled breathing and selective attention. By focusing on your body, you leave those negative thoughts behind that maintain anxiety and stress. This is much more effective than simply trying to ignore those thoughts or attempting to resolve them. The former only reinforces the thoughts; the latter only works on very specific problems that are within your control.

Suitability

When we feel under threat, our focus is on the threat in front of us. If the threat is more abstract, then we focus on our thoughts in an attempt to circumvent the threat before it occurs or intensifies. Unfortunately, this preoccupation with our thoughts can make us feel worse. Body Scan provides an alternative solution to dealing with distressful situations, by guiding us to focus on our breathing and bodily sensations. This makes it suitable for anyone experiencing overwhelming emotions. I don't recommend it for people with health anxiety or panic disorder, as the further focusing on the body might aggravate your negative symptoms rather than reduce them.

How to use

Focus on your lungs and their expansion and contraction as you slow your breathing down and take deeper breaths. If you feel comfortable, close your eyes. Now turn your attention towards your feet. As you breathe, how do they feel? Press your feet into the ground and spread your toes. In your mind, try to describe any sensations that you feel. Picture your breath travelling from your lungs down to your feet. Then add to this process and imagine your breath running through your calves, your thighs and your stomach. If there is any tightness, release it. Try to rid yourself of any uncomfortableness or constriction.

Now add the rest of your limbs to the exercise. Tell yourself that your breath is freeing your body from tension, like a strong wind blowing away the cobwebs in an attic. Visualise that tension flowing upwards out of the top of your head, then being expelled and dispersing into the void. When you notice that your emotions are not as overwhelming as before, count to three, open your eyes and return to the world. Use the space provided in the worksheet to note any reflections you may have after using this technique.

Body Scan

- Bring your awareness to your chest and to your breathing. Close your eyes
- Notice the sensations in your feet. Imagine that your breath is flowing in and out from the bottom of your soles
- Now focus attention on your ankles and calves and how the flow of your breath runs through them
- Bring attention to your other body parts. Let go of any sensations that constrict and limit
- Focus on any parts of your body that carry tension and imagine your breath moving to those spaces
- Picture a hole at the top of your head and allow your breath to redirect any discomfort or pain through that hole
- On a count of three, return to your surroundings. Open your eyes. Feel any changes

Reflections

I imagined my breath travelling through my body and purifying all those worries and doubts about the future. I tried to stay in the present and picture the steps. The powerful image of a blowhole at the top of my head, where all those doubts escaped, helped my focus and prevented my mind from retreating back on itself.

3.5 Mundane Task Focusing

Mohlman, J. (2004). Attention training as an intervention for anxiety: Review and rationale. *The Behavior Therapist, 27*(2), 37–41.

Purpose

Some people don't like relaxation exercises. Sometimes focusing on breathing or on tense muscles actually increases their anxiety. This can be demotivating and discourage them from gaining the benefits of redirecting attention. Mundane task focusing is a novel way of redirecting your attention away from your thoughts. Instead of focusing on your body and breathing, the worksheet encourages you to turn your attention towards mundane tasks that engage your senses.

We have all experienced that trance-like state when we are doing something rhythmic that requires little mental energy but keeps our attention fixed on the task in front of us. These mundane tasks can be employed to therapeutic ends. When you next find your attention wandering towards a catastrophic future or a regret-filled past, use this worksheet to redirect your mind elsewhere. The relief you get may be temporary, but you can then explore what this tells you about how your mind holds on to negative thoughts.

Suitability

People with health anxiety or panic disorder may find this exercise helps them reduce the need to check their body for signs of ill health. Similarly, people who are hypersensitive to noise might find that repeating a mundane task will help them distance themselves from the feelings provoked by the intrusive sounds. Concentration is one of the first things to suffer when we have a lot on our mind, so use Mundane Task Focusing to train your attention in the same way you would train a muscle to improve its endurance.

How to use

First, write a list of mundane tasks that you do on a daily basis. These can be routine chores that you do around the house and ideally should involve some sort of movement and co-ordination. The emphasis should be on activities that require little energy and that are already well integrated into your life. Then put the worksheet away until you next find your mind wandering and your anxiety levels increasing.

When this occurs, record on the worksheet what percentage of your attention is on your anxious thoughts and what percentage is on the activity you were engaged in. In total they should add up to 100%.

Next, engage in one of your chosen mundane tasks. Do whichever task is most convenient for you at the time. When performing the task, focus on your senses. What do you feel with your hands when you are folding your clothes? What does the fresh laundry smell like? If you feel your anxious thoughts encroaching again, gently redirect your attention towards what you are experiencing in the present. If you are doing something that has a natural rhythm, such as brushing your teeth or washing the dishes, it can sometimes help to count every stroke. It is difficult to count and simultaneously worry or ruminate, so use this to your advantage and allow the counting to moderate any intense, distracting thoughts.

When you have finished the mundane task, score again how your attention was divided. Hopefully you should see that, when you had a purposeful task in mind, your attention was less self-orientated and more focused on the task in front of you. Consider what that says about your straying thoughts and spiralling doubts and worries. Are they, in fact, as uncontrollable as you thought?

Mundane Task Focusing

Mundane tasks
Brushing my teeth
Doing the laundry
Polishing my shoes
Cleaning the dishes
Cleaning the windows
Weeding the garden

Self-focused attention	70 %
Task-focused attention	30 %

Engage in chosen mundane task: if attention wanders, focus on all five senses

Self-focused attention	40 %
Task-focused attention	60 %

3.6 Grounding

Fisher, J. (1999). *The work of stabilization in trauma treatment.* Paper presented at the Trauma Center Lecture Series, 1999. Boston, MA. https://janinafisher.com/pdfs/stabilize.pdf

Purpose

Anxiety is often maintained by a preoccupation with our thoughts. We catastrophise, imagine worst-case scenarios and allow negative thoughts to come upon us, one after another. This process can be interrupted in many ways. Grounding introduces the idea that, by turning your attention towards your senses, you can give yourself a break from overthinking and get back in touch with the present. When you start naming everything that your senses can distinguish, you draw a line between what is in front of you, what is in your past and what your future might contain. When your attention is grounded in the present, it becomes much easier to see the past and future as remote. This might not make the thoughts go away entirely, but it can reduce their emotional intensity.

Suitability

All relaxation strategies involve centring yourself in the present. Grounding achieves this by getting you to tune into your senses and list what you experience. This is particularly helpful if you are having frequent flashbacks to the past and feel you are reliving traumatic memories. By naming what your senses pick up, you can find it easier to stay in the present and distinguish what is in the past. Ultimately, this is a technique that redirects your attention away from your thoughts and towards the reality of the environment around you. It is suitable for anyone experiencing anxiety, but people with PTSD should find it especially helpful as it can be used alongside other experimental models in this book that might increase your anxiety.

How to use

When you feel anxiety or panic beginning to form, take out this worksheet and follow its instructions. Start by naming five things you can see. You can name them out loud or in your head, whichever you are more comfortable with. Then name four things that you can feel. These can be things that you are touching right now, or you can reach out and brush your hands against other surfaces. Next, name three things that you can hear. Sometimes it can be quite tough to distinguish between individual sounds. If you have trouble doing so, keep in mind that you can always create a sound by (say) rubbing your feet against the ground. Then name two smells. Again, it might be difficult to put a name to any smells, but this is not necessarily a terrible thing. The more your mind struggles to identify and name a particular sensory experience, the less energy it has to expend on your anxious thoughts. Finally, name one thing that you can taste.

Once you are done, check on your anxiety. Has it decreased? If it is still quite intense, repeat the exercise. Feel free to swap out some of the sensations for others, if they have changed. Keep this process going until your anxiety is back at a reasonable level and you feel you can continue with your daily life. Use the space provided on this worksheet to add any reflections that have occurred to you. The more you use this worksheet, the easier and quicker it should become to manage your anxiety levels.

Grounding

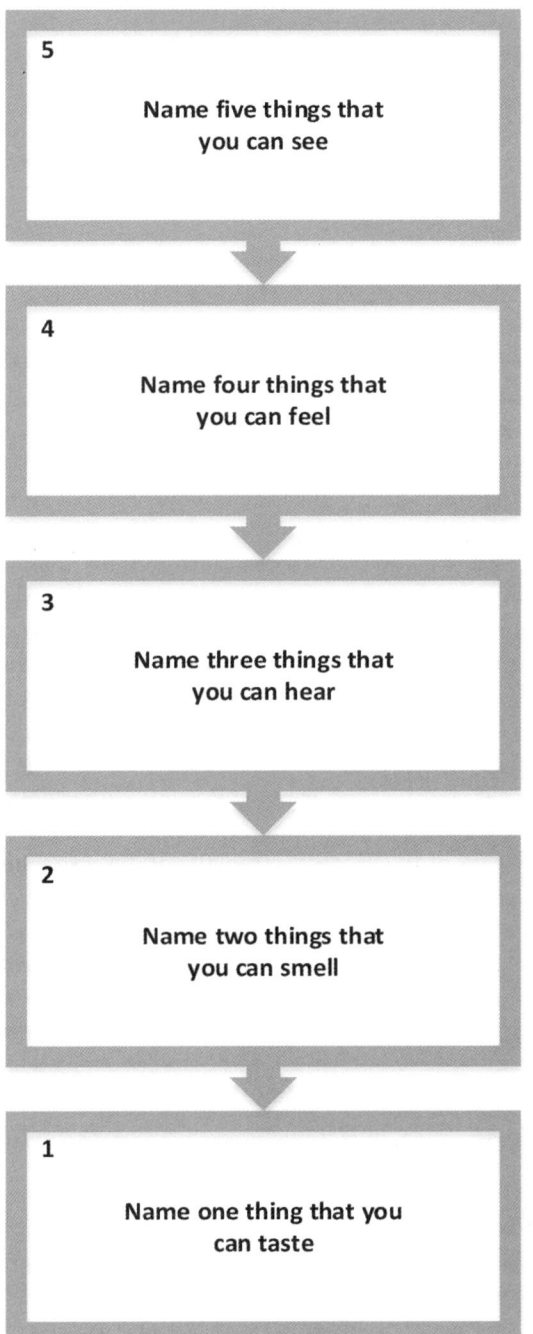

Reflections

I tried to ground myself whenever intrusive thoughts entered my head this week. When I was alone, I said each of the things that I could sense out loud. Seeing and feeling was easy enough, but as I progressed down the list it became harder and I had to search for things longer. It was a challenge putting words to what I smelled, but I think searching my vocabulary took my mind off what was making me so anxious. Doing this exercise really made me conscious of where I was and what was around me. I felt a little safer and more secure because of it. I intend to keep practising this as it was easy to do and only took a minute to complete.

Chapter 4. Diary-keeping

Introduction

Journalling is widely regarded as therapeutic. Allocating time at the end of a busy day to reflect on recent events and how you are feeling can give you perspective and the opportunity to consider any obstacles in your way. This chapter is primarily concerned with diary-keeping, but for specific purposes. Writing down your thoughts in an unstructured manner can allow you to engage in a dialogue with yourself, but the diaries here are also concerned with highlighting the persistent difficulties in your life that remain resistant to change. This is in line with the CBT principle of specificity: that every individual problem needs an individual solution. It would quickly become overwhelming if you tried to complete all these diaries at once. Instead, you should focus on one at a time, choosing the diary that best matches your requirements.

Many of the diaries focus on recording the specific situations that cause you distress. This might be because the situation makes you anxious about your health (Health Anxiety Thought Record, p.80), results in problematic behaviour (Problematic Behaviour Diary, p.72) or leads to intrusive thoughts (Intrusive Thoughts Diary, p.84). They follow a similar pattern: they highlight the situation, your thoughts, behaviours and emotions, and then encourage some form of interpretation. For instance, if you are completing the Worry Diary (p.70), you will be asked to reflect on whether your worries are unimportant, important and can be solved, or important and cannot be solved. This is designed to encourage you to re-examine what you have control over and what is outside your control. One of the greatest strengths of diary-keeping is that, the more entries you add, the more evidence accumulates and the easier it becomes to see where you might be regularly misinterpreting situations.

Other diaries in this chapter put emphasis on what you have done well. If you become more aware that certain sleeping patterns improve your day, or certain activities make you feel closer to others and less depressed, then you can begin to map the line from those positive outcomes to your preceding behaviours and thoughts. This can dispel the idea that you feel better on certain days for no reason at all. Instead, it might be because you are unconsciously putting in place helpful coping devices. Diaries such as the Panic Diary (p.78) or Food Journal (p.76) can help you realise how many almost imperceptible factors influence how you feel.

You will notice that many of the diaries involve rating how you feel or how much you believe in something. This highlights another feature of diary-keeping: namely, that it serves as a way to track progress. If, for example, you are working your way through the OCD Ritual Diary (p.86) and recording every time you complete a ritual to rid yourself of a compulsion, you will be encouraged to write down the level of discomfort that you feel on a scale of 0–100. If you then combine your diary-keeping with some of the thought-challenging exercises in Chapter 5, you should start to see that your levels of discomfort slowly decrease as your belief in the effectiveness of the rituals wanes. Keeping a diary can make you aware of this, while also indicating when progress is not being made and you should try another strategy.

For diary-keeping to be truly effective, it needs to be integrated with other therapeutic practices. If you have set out to master the relaxation strategies in the previous chapter, reflect whether it would be helpful to use the Relaxation Diary (p.74) as a way to measure their effectiveness. While the models in this book are organised by theme, I recommend that you approach them in a non-linear fashion, range across them freely and allow your preferences and needs to dictate how you combine them.

A question that sometimes arises is how long you should keep a diary for, and when, if ever, you should swap over to another. I recommend that you focus your energy on the diary that currently mirrors the nature of your difficulties most accurately, and continue until that is no longer the case. Then you can decide whether to add another diary or stop diary-keeping altogether. In the meantime, use diary-keeping as a way to identify and refine your most pressing issues.

4.1 Worry Diary

Dugas, M.J. & Robichaud, M. (2007). *Cognitive behavioral treatment for generalized anxiety disorder.* Routledge.

Purpose

If the first step towards reducing anxiety is awareness of your worries, it makes sense to record them using a diary so you can better recollect their nature and frequency. This allows you to track your progress more effectively and distinguish more clearly the types of worry. This is an important component of worry management, as the therapeutic path you next take depends on the type of worries you have.

The Worry Diary is a tool that not only allows you to record your worries but also helps you understand which worries are within your control and can be solved and which are not and therefore you are powerless to solve. The difference this can make is profound. If you are using all your energy and time trying to solve what cannot be solved, your stress levels and anxiety will quickly become unmanageable.

Suitability

The Worry Diary is suitable for anyone experiencing frequent worries who struggles to separate those that are within their control from those that are not. People who have generalised anxiety disorder (GAD) will find this model particularly useful, as often the sheer number of different worries can be overwhelming, and it is difficult to keep track of them all. The Worry Diary should quickly reveal whether your next step in treatment is to work on problem-solving (Cost/Benefit Analysis, Chapter 5, p.98) or on hypothetical worry management (Worry Time, Chapter 6, p.120).

How to use

Use the diary to record the worries you experience during the week. It can be helpful to keep the diary close to hand as you go through the day, so you can immediately note down any worries that occur. If you are out and about, you could use your phone to record your worries so you don't miss any. The Worry Diary asks you to write down the situation you find yourself in when your worry surfaces, then capture the specific thoughts that come to mind and their significance to you. Ask yourself what it is that you fear might happen and what emotions are triggered by these thoughts.

Once you have grounded your worry by recording these details, classify it as one of three types. The first type are the unimportant worries. These are worries about things that, even if the worst were to happen, would not be overly upsetting. They might be very fleeting, which it is why it is all the more important to record them when they are present. The second are worries that are important and can be solved in the immediate future. They must include solutions that are within your control to implement and that you can easily measure. The final type are worries that are important but you cannot solve them. These are sometimes referred to as hypothetical worries as they involve your mind imagining scenarios that present little actual threat in the present but, were they to happen, would have disastrous results.

The greatest challenge with classifying your worries is recognising what can be solved and what cannot. It is tempting to see hypothetical worries as solvable if you stay hypervigilant to threats, prepare for the worst and see the act of worrying as necessary to stay safe. This approach might give you an illusion of control, but it will also maintain your worry while not resolving any of your difficulties.

Worry Diary

Situation	Thoughts	What do you fear might happen?	Emotions	Not important	Important and can be solved	Important but cannot be solved
At the supermarket	What if I buy something that we already have in the cupboards?	That I will end up with more of something than I need	Annoyance, doubt	X		
Looking through a stack of bills at home	If I lose my job, I will not be able to afford to pay these bills.	That I will become homeless and destitute	Nervousness, on edge, fear			X
Noticing the car is running out of petrol	If we run out of petrol we might end up stranded	Having to call for help	Embarrassment, trepidation		X	

4.2 Problematic Behaviour Diary

Day, A., Howells, K., Mohr, P., Schall, E., & Gerace, A. (2008). The development of CBT programmes for anger: The role of interventions to promote perspective-taking skills. *Behavioural and Cognitive Psychotherapy, 36*(3), 299–312.

Purpose

Problematic behaviour can be defined as behaviour that has negative consequences for you or for others. Much problematic behaviour is incentivised by either short-term pleasure or a sense of release. Nevertheless, in the long-term, this behaviour causes more problems than it solves. While it can be a challenge to identify your problematic behaviours, as what is problematic for one person can be a healthy coping strategy for another, there are some behaviours that seem to consistently result in poor outcomes.

The first step to dealing with problematic behaviour is to record it when it happens. A Problematic Behaviour Diary can capture these situations and provide some awareness of the consequences of your actions. It can then be used to imagine hypothetical scenarios where you act differently. Hopefully this will demonstrate that you are not trapped by your behaviours but can in fact use them, alongside a change in thinking, to escape your destructive cycles.

Suitability

By focusing on behaviour, the Problematic Behaviour Diary allows you to reflect on what defines problematic behaviour and explore possible alternative behaviours. It does so by emphasising the consequences of the behaviour. If a particular act has unpleasant consequences and you become more aware of the repercussions, you will, it stands to reason, be more motivated to stop doing it. This model can be used by anyone, but people who self-harm, have addiction problems or pursue risky behaviour might find it particularly helpful.

How to use

Begin the week with the intention of recording any problematic behaviour that you might engage in. As the days go by, record these instances and describe the situation you were in and the consequences of your behaviour. The consequences can be how you felt or how others reacted towards you. They can follow your actions immediately or their true import might only become clearer near the end of the day.

As you record these incidents, ask yourself what you could have done differently. If, instead of isolating yourself from your family when you felt low, you had made the effort to talk to them and offered to help them, would that have had different consequences? Write down what you think might have happened and then reflect on what that tells you about your emotional state, the role of your behaviours or any other psychological observations that come to mind. Use those reflections to inspire further alternative new behaviours.

Problematic Behaviour Diary

Trigger	Behaviour	Consequences of behaviour	Potential new behaviour	Potential new consequences of behaviour	Reflection
Was late for a job interview	I was flustered during the interview and I spoke very fast and wasn't very clear	I think it might have cost me the job	To remind myself that sometimes people are late. Breathe	I seem calmer and more confident in future interviews	That I have control over how I come across to others
Got into argument with partner about household chores	Yelled and shouted and then left the house to get fresh air	My partner and I were not on good terms for the rest of the week	Not leaving the house when angry	My partner and I are more open with one another	Avoidance is not a long-term solution
My football team lost an important game	Hit my head against the wall several times	It gave me a headache and I felt really foolish and ashamed of myself	To put the loss into perspective	I won't become so self-critical of my behaviour	I should try not to release my emotions with violent behaviour

4.3 Relaxation Diary

Barlow, D.H. (2004). *Anxiety and its disorders: The nature and treatment of anxiety and panic.* Guilford Press.

Purpose

Relaxation techniques reduce anxiety by redirecting our attention away from perceived threats and towards our breathing or other calming actions. However, while these techniques can be very effective once learned, obstacles can sometimes arise that prevent you from fully internalising the lessons that they teach.

A Relaxation Diary can help you keep track of your attempts to put into practice specific relaxation techniques. This can help with motivation and adherence. The diary can also help you monitor the effectiveness of the techniques. Seeing your anxiety decrease is evidence in itself, but being able to look back in a diary and see that each entry over several weeks confirms how selective attention reduces negative emotions is a remarkably powerful testament to your abilities and the powers of relaxation. Furthermore, the diary can demonstrate progress. You will quite quickly find that it takes less and less time to practise the techniques. You should also find that the number of times your anxiety reaches peaks such that the diary is needed reduces quickly too. All of this should indicate your increased competence in managing intense emotions.

Suitability

Anyone who experiences anxiety should find the Relaxation Diary helpful. It will give you a better understanding of how and which relaxation exercises can help reduce the intensity of your emotions and strength of the negative physical symptoms. Recording the instances where you confront your anxiety will give you evidence of your own efficacy in using these techniques. Once you have seen what you can do simply by redirecting your attention, this should inspire you with the confidence to meet other challenges.

How to use

The Relaxation Diary should be used alongside the relaxation techniques described in Chapter 3. Start by learning a couple of the relaxation techniques well enough that you don't need to consult the book. When you next feel anxious, test out one of these techniques to reduce the intensity of your feelings. Once you feel more in control, record in the diary the situation and the relaxation technique you used.

Now think back and score your initial anxiety on a scale of 0–100. Then note approximately how long you spent doing the relaxation exercise. Finish by recording your current anxiety levels after using the relaxation technique, using the same scoring system. Hopefully you should see a significant decrease between the two scores. The greater the decrease, the more effective and appropriate the relaxation technique.

As the days go by, continue to record your use of the relaxation techniques. Look out for the following: is there a consistent pattern showing a decrease in anxiety when you use the techniques? Do any particular techniques seem more effective than others? Is there a decrease in the time it takes for you to perform the techniques? These questions can offer further insight to the effectiveness of using selective attention to reduce anxiety.

Relaxation Diary

Situation	Anxiety before %	Relaxation technique	Time spent using technique	Anxiety after %
Wednesday, 13:00: deadline coming up at work	70%	Square breathing	3mins	50%
Friday, 17:00: getting ready for a date	80%	Mindfulness meditation	5mins	40%
Sunday, 11:00: trying to figure out how to use a website to order a gift	50%	Progressive muscle relaxation	8mins	40%

4.4 Food Journal

Fairburn, C.G. (2008). *Cognitive behavior therapy and eating disorders*. Guilford Press.

Purpose

Our mental health is vulnerable to many factors. Stressful life events, overthinking, unhealthy coping devices, toxic working or living environments – all of these and more can impact how we feel and behave. While we are all aware that eating too much can lead to obesity and eating too little can cause other physical health conditions, we do not always realise how essential a healthy diet and regular eating patterns are to our mental wellbeing

Using a food journal to reflect on our eating habits can make us realise when we are eating too much or too little; that the food choices we are making are poor, and that these decisions may intensify any negative emotional states we are already in. Food, for example, is sometimes used as a coping device to reduce short-term anxiety, but doing so can lead to feelings of guilt and worthlessness. Too much caffeine or sugar can have an adverse effect on anxiety, and if you are eating too little, you will not have the energy to engage in activities that can reduce your depression. Nevertheless, we often overlook regular eating times and proper nutrition when we are trying manage mental distress. Using a food journal can address these issues and ensure that you become more conscious of any unhelping eating patterns you may have.

Suitability

Anyone can use the Food Journal to begin to explore their relationship with food and how it might intersect with their mental health. If you have already noticed symptoms such as loss of appetite or comfort eating, then I recommend you use this journal to track any developments in these areas. However, while keeping a food journal can be a good start to exploring and managing eating disorders, it is not enough on its own. Seek professional help if you are concerned that you have a more complex relationship with food.

How to use

At the end of each day, record what you have eaten and drunk. The structure of the journal divides your meals into breakfast, lunch, dinner and snacks. Not everyone will naturally follow this meal routine, and the journal will show how far you deviate from it. For instance, if you are always skipping breakfast and lunch, that might cause low energy at the start of the day and lead you to snacking all day or eating too much in the evening. Explore how your eating patterns reflect your moods. Do you feel more anxious at a certain time of day, and could that be partially attributed to low blood sugar after a sugar high has worn off? Do you feel sleepy after eating certain foods in the middle of the day?

There is additional space to record what you have drunk through the day. This will show you what sugar, caffeine or calories you might be consuming in drinks. Often, we forget to account for drinks when tallying up our day's consumption. Watch out for any signs of dehydration, as a lot of unpleasant physical symptoms can be attributed to not drinking enough water. Another factor to watch out for is irritability if you are drinking a lot of coffee. And remember that coffee and tea are of themselves dehydrating, so you do need to keep drinking plain water as well. Excess alcohol is, of course, not good for our mental or physical health, and most alcoholic drinks contain a lot of calories.

At the end of the week, look back at what you have written and consider what might need changing. If there are several issues that need work, start a fresh Food Journal and plan out a healthier food and drink schedule for the coming week. Then monitor it, using the diary to help you stick to that plan.

Food Journal

	Monday	Tuesday	Wednesday	Thursday	Friday	Saturday	Sunday
Breakfast	N/A	Cereal with milk, apple	Weetabix with milk, banana	N/A	Omelette with tomatoes	Cereal with milk, apple	Bacon, eggs, baked beans, mushrooms
Lunch	Two ham and cheese sandwiches	N/A	Chicken panini	Vegetarian wrap and blueberry muffin	N/A	N/A	N/A
Dinner	Chicken korma curry with rice and naan bread	Stir fry with noodles and prawns	Instant noodles	Fast food burger and fries, with ice cream afterwards	Steak, potatoes, spinach	Salmon, asparagus, rice	Lasagne
Snacks	Bag of crisps	Chocolate bar	Bag of nuts	N/A	Two packets of crisps, kebab	Half a cheesecake	N/A
Drinks	Two soft drinks, one coffee, 0.5 litres of water	One coffee, 1 litre of water	One coffee, two teas, 0.5 litres of water	One coffee, one soft drink, 1 litre of water	Three glasses of wine, one coffee	One glass of wine, two coffees, 0.5 litres of water	One coffee, one hot chocolate, 1.5 litres of water

4.5 Panic Diary

Barlow, D.H. & Craske, M.G. (2006). *Mastery of your anxiety and panic.* Oxford University Press.

Purpose

Panic attacks can strike without notice and leave us feeling dizzy, nauseous and gasping for air. They are a very distressing experience and seemingly outside our control. However, if we can identify triggers, recognise patterns in our coping behaviours and challenge our initial explanations for why they are occurring, we can take back some of that control.

A Panic Diary allows you to record your panic attacks and gain a little more clarity over their nature. It is important here to remind yourself that, no matter how intense a panic attack becomes, it will not cause you lasting harm. Recording your panic attacks and exposing yourself to anxiety-inducing situations will not put you in danger. The opposite, in fact, will occur, as you become more aware that you can control your anxiety by, for example, using relaxation techniques and revising your explanations for the panic attacks.

If you tell yourself that every time you get a panic attack you may end up in hospital, this is anxiety inducing in its own right, and will make your anxiety worse, not better. If you can counter such thoughts with more rational responses, you will have a better chance of managing the intensity of the panic attack far more successfully.

Suitability

The Panic Diary is a useful tool for anyone experiencing regular panic attacks. It enables you to easily record them and describe them in detail. It also provides a reality check between what you fear might happen and what actually happens. This can help you come up with alternative explanations for why the panic attacks occur and what actually causes your symptoms to abate. I suggest you keep a record of how many panic attacks you have every week; together, that record and this worksheet are an excellent way of measuring your progress and the reduction in number and intensity of your panic attacks.

How to use

Start with the intention of recording every panic attack you experience. Ensure that you identify the situation that triggers the panic and the physical symptoms. Score the intensity of those symptoms on a scale of 0–100. Note down your feared consequences in the moment. What significance did you give your symptoms? Did you think you were having a heart attack or were the symptoms less severe?

Describe your behaviour when you were feeling at your worst. How did you make the panic symptoms go away? Sometimes we feel we have no control over our symptoms; at other times our coping strategies may seem to reduce the intensity of our panic. It can be beneficial to also record what the actual consequences of the panic were. If you start to catastrophise every time you have a panic attack, these recurring observations might convince you that the worst-case scenarios, such as heart attack, fainting and even death, will not happen.

Finally, record an alternative explanation for your symptoms. This is where you apply your understanding of anxiety, the fight/flight response and selective attention. Hopefully you are by now at least partially convinced that panic is often just a misinterpretation of a threat that our thoughts and behaviours over time reinforce and maintain.

Panic Diary

Situation	Intensity %	Physical symptoms	Feared consequences	Behaviour	Actual consequences	Alternative explanation
Riding on the metro	80%	Sweaty palms, racing heart, shallow breathing	I will pass out	I got off the train at the next stop	I did not suffocate	By focusing on my symptoms I made the anxiety worse
Walking home at night	70%	Heart palpitations, difficulty breathing	I am in danger. I can't keep myself safe	I ran home	I was not attacked	The flight/fight response took over
Running late for an appointment	40%	Racing thoughts, fast breathing, headache	I will be late and I will be judged negatively	I hurried and felt stressed the whole trip	My colleague did not notice that I was late	I tried to mind-read what my colleague would think of me
Worrying about the debt I am in when going over my bills	60%	Felt dizzy, fast breathing	I will be homeless. I can't handle all the stress	I stopped looking at the bills and went out the room	I still have a home	I caused my body to react negatively from thought alone

4.6 Health Anxiety Thought Record

Taylor, S. (2005). Understanding and treating health anxiety: A cognitive-behavioral approach. *Cognitive and Behavioral Practice, 11*(1), 112–123.

Purpose

The purpose behind using a Health Anxiety Thought Record is to help you understand what causes and maintains health anxiety. It allows you to apply your psychological knowledge towards discovering a more rational explanation for why the anxiety occurs in the first place. Having done this, you should be better equipped to deal with future situations where health anxiety might arise.

Health anxiety is the firm belief that your health is in jeopardy. You begin to see your body as a threat – that the only way to stay safe is to remain constantly hypervigilant, checking your body for new symptoms, calling your doctor for advice or researching explanations for your symptoms on the internet. These strategies might reduce your anxiety temporarily, but this in itself reinforces the belief that you need to stay vigilant and seek more and more information and support. The only way to end this cycle is to realise that your negative physical symptoms and emotional states are not the result of a health condition but are the product of being constantly on guard against danger.

Suitability

Keeping a Healthy Anxiety Thought Record is useful for people with frequent, unfounded anxieties about their health. People with actual health conditions who think they may be disproportionately anxious about them may also find it helpful, as may those who have not been diagnosed with any underlying health condition but still believe that they are facing a physical health crisis.

How to use

Begin by recording the times during the day that you feel anxious about your health. Describe the specific context. What was happening at the time the anxiety emerged? Were there any noticeable triggers that brought on the negative thoughts? Describe how the thought made you feel and how you reacted to it. You may have redirected your attention, sought reassurance or isolated yourself from others. This is important to note as, in the long term, some of these behaviours can maintain health anxiety, even while they provide the illusion of being the cure to your problems.

The final section of the thought record asks you to provide a more rational response to the negative thought. This can be quite challenging, as it requires you to take a more objective view of what you are experiencing. It might be too much to ask while you are feeling everything so intensely. If that is the case, give yourself some space before investigating alternative explanations that might better explain how you feel.

When exploring other, more rational alternatives, keep in mind how anxiety is maintained by selective attention to perceived threats. If you are excessively focusing on your body, on a tragic news story or on distressing thoughts about the past, your anxiety is bound to increase, alongside a number of unpleasant physical symptoms. Be sure to question whether those symptoms are from an undiagnosed health condition or are actually a side-effect of your anxiety.

Health Anxiety Thought Record

Date/time	Trigger	Emotion	Negative thought	How I responded	Rational response to negative thought
15/07/2022	Running for the bus	Fear	I'm breathing too hard, something must be wrong	I took my phone out in case I had to call for an ambulance	That my breathing was a result of my exertion, not from any underlying health condition
15/07/2022	Doing the laundry	Anger, confusion, fear	Why am I getting heart palpitations? It must be bad	I called my partner and they reassured me	Sometimes physical symptoms have a psychological cause. Not everything is rooted in my body
16/07/2022	Watching the news on TV	Concern, exhaustion, fear	So much is going wrong... just like with my health	I started examining my body	The more I look for problems, the more I will find. The act of looking can increase anxiety
17/07/2022	Having a conversation about my operation	Anxiety, sadness, trepidation	I started noticing a ringing in my ears. New symptom!	I focused on the ringing and then researched it on my computer	If I have conversations about my health, my attention will be redirected to my body and my anxiety will increase

4.7 Critical Voice Record

Gilbert, P. (2005). Compassion and cruelty: A biopsychosocial approach. In P. Gilbert (Ed.), *Compassion: Conceptualisations, research and use in psychotherapy* (pp.9–74). Routledge.

Purpose

We all have an inner voice that comments on and narrates our inner life. This voice can be our best friend and can motivate us to overcome obstacles and fight our fears. However, it can also be our worst enemy and undermine our progress. When we have been feeling low for many months or years, our inner voice can become overly critical. Where before you might have seen an opportunity, now all you see is potential for failure. Ambiguous situations suddenly become negative as you listen to that critical voice and take what it says for granted.

A Critical Voice Record can help us challenge these negative thoughts and balance them with more compassionate alternatives. This is not to force you to see everything in a positive light. Rather, it is about helping you see that most situations or self-appraisals can be distorted by our mood and habits. If we are having a terrible day, we are more likely to judge ourselves more harshly if something else unpleasant happens. Moreover, if we have got into the habit of speaking to ourselves in a particularly negative way, new situations might not even warrant such critical thoughts, but we think them all the same. The purpose of this record is to break those old habits and introduce new ones that may be of more benefit to our mental health.

Suitability

Many forms of depression include a lot of self-criticism. If you think this applies to you, consider using the Critical Voice Record to list these thoughts and present more self-compassionate ways of speaking to yourself.

How to use

Every time you have a critical thought about yourself, write it down on the worksheet. Describe the situation you were in and the emotions you felt at the time. Then score your belief in the critical thought box on a scale of 0–100. The higher you score the thought, the harder it will be to imagine thinking in any other way. Hopefully none of your scores reaches 100, as that would suggest a belief that things can never change. If any beliefs do score that high, consider going back to the record when your emotions are less intense. Perhaps then you will be able to be a little kinder to yourself.

After grading your belief in the self-critical thought, try to imagine a more self-compassionate alternative. This doesn't have to be something you believe in. It is fine simply to write what you imagine another person would experience in the same situation. What can sometimes help with this is to imagine a friend came to you with the same self-critical thought – how would you convince them that they were partially or entirely mistaken? Often we judge others much less severely than we do ourselves.

By the end of the week, you should have a record of all your self-critical thoughts and more compassionate alternatives. No doubt many of the same self-doubts and critical thoughts will reappear in coming weeks. If that happens, remind yourself of those self-compassionate alternatives and see if that reduces, if only slightly, the intensity of the negative emotions and the strength of the self-critical thought.

Critical Voice Record

Situation	Self-critical thought	Emotion	Belief in critical thought %	Self-compassionate alternative thought
I failed to get into the university I wanted	I'm a terrible student. Why do I bother? I'm no good at academic work	Sadness, defeat, frustration	80%	I have got into other universities. A lot of my friends didn't get their first choice either
My friend cancelled our tennis game	I'm not a good enough player to offer them a challenge. They'd rather play with others	Disappointment, inadequacy	60%	People play tennis with me not because of how good I am, but because they enjoy my company
My brother just bought a new car	I can't afford to buy a car. I'm never going to be able to make that kind of money	Jealousy, low self-esteem	75%	My brother is a lot older than me and I have plenty of time to catch up with him

4.8 Intrusive Thoughts Diary

Wells, A. (1997). *Cognitive therapy of anxiety disorders: A practice manual and conceptual guide.* John Wiley & Sons.

Purpose

Intrusive thoughts are thoughts that come to us seemingly from nowhere and feel near-impossible to divert. They can often involve a fear of some great disaster or mistake that, if not immediately corrected, will lead to harm coming to you or your loved ones. These thoughts can be very distressing, more so because we feel responsible for whether the imagined disaster occurs or not. As there is such a burden on us to act, our behaviours too take on great significance. We must make sure that anything we do to keep ourselves safe is done perfectly, even if it that involves doing it over and over again.

What I've just described is the thought and behaviour process behind obsessive-compulsive disorder (OCD). An Intrusive Thoughts Diary is designed to help us to identify those specific types of thoughts, the meaning we give them and the behaviours that we believe keep us safe. The purpose of such recording is to allow us to see how our thoughts and behaviours become obsessions and compulsions. Once we've realised this, we can seek to change our thinking patterns, and so improve the quality of our lives.

Suitability

The Intrusive Thoughts Diary is intended for people with symptoms of OCD. Many of us have intrusive thoughts, but this diary is concerned with the specific meanings we attribute to those thoughts (obsessions) and the role our behaviour (compulsions) has in reducing the intensity of how we feel. The diary preludes the cognitive restructuring techniques in Chapter 5, such as Unhelpful Thinking styles (Chapter 5, p.92) and the Thought-Disputing Model (Chapter 5, p.94), and I suggest you follow it eventually with OCD Graded Exposure (Chapter 6, p.132).

How to use

Write down any intrusive thoughts that enter your head. Ensure that you record the situation you are in and any significant triggers that arose. Next, write down the significance of the intrusive thoughts to you. What makes them recur and why is it so difficult to refocus your attention elsewhere? When you interpret the meaning of your thoughts, think about any worst-case scenarios or catastrophic thinking styles that you might be adopting.

Then move on to describe your behaviour in response to these thoughts. How do you ensure that the intrusive thoughts do not come true? Often the behaviour can seem to cleanse us of the dangers of our thoughts. We think that, if we repeat an activity enough times, what we imagine won't come to pass. These rituals provide an illusion of safety, but in fact can only reduce your anxiety. This is a key difference that, once you understand it, can release you from the tyranny of obsessive rumination.

Intrusive Thoughts Diary

Trigger/situation	Intrusive thought	Interpretation of intrusive thought	Behaviour to reduce intensity of intrusive thought
Entering the house and closing the door behind me	If I don't lock the door, someone could break in easily	I am responsible for my own security and safety and that of my family	Checking several times to see if the door is locked
Washing the dishes	If the dishes aren't clean they could cause food poisoning next time they are used	If I don't clean the dishes properly, I could make someone really ill	Washing each dish several times
Praying in the evening	If I miss out someone in my prayers, some misfortune might happen to them	I need to make sure that everybody is included or something terrible could happen	Repeating my prayers several times
Cooking for my family	If I don't turn off the oven, the house might catch fire	It is only my hypervigilance that keeps my family and house safe	Constantly checking that the oven is turned off

4.9 OCD Ritual Diary

Wells, A. (1997). *Cognitive therapy of anxiety disorders: A practice manual and conceptual guide.* John Wiley & Sons.

Purpose

A defining characteristic of obsessive-compulsive disorder (OCD) is an urge to enact specific ritualistic behaviours in order to reduce the intensity of obsessions. Bringing awareness to this fact, OCD Ritual Diary allows you to measure the discomfort you feel before performing your ritual, and then the length of time you spend engaged in it. This should provide you with the means to track your progress as you begin to decouple the idea that these specific compulsions are connected with holding back imminent disaster.

The purpose behind diary-keeping is to give yourself a more accurate picture of what you are doing during the day. Often we minimise or magnify certain behaviours and imagine that we are doing more or less of them than is actually the case. These distortions can be harmful as they can aggravate existing difficulties, either by brushing them under the carpet or by giving them undue significance. You may think that your OCD behaviour does not last that long, but when you look at a clock, it will tell you exactly how long you have spent performing your rituals. This is time that you could be spending doing the things you love.

Suitability

Anyone who has OCD will benefit from a greater understanding of their ritualistic behaviour. Keeping a diary that identifies the triggering situation, the ritual and its intensity and duration will help you measure the severity of your condition and whether your attempts to reduce your OCD behaviours have been successful. Positive evidence can further motivate you to continue with your efforts. This diary can be used alongside Intrusive Thoughts Diary (p.84) as together they deal with the twin poles of OCD: obsessions and compulsions.

How to use

Focus on recording any rituals that you perform during the week. Note down the situation you are in and describe the nature of the ritual. Score on a scale of 0–100 the discomfort you felt before you started performing the ritual. Then record the time you spent performing the ritual. If you have a specific ritual that you repeat several times, be sure to add up the total time you spend doing it. The diary may quickly fill up. Do not be put off by this. The point of this diary is to highlight the frequency and repetitive nature of your behaviour, so it stands to reason that the diary entries will begin to mount up.

So, continue with the diary, as hopefully you should start to see small signs of progress. Maybe you'll find you are spending less time ritually cleaning the house, or you feel less discomfort when you go out without double-checking you've locked the front door. As you discover that your ritualistic behaviour only temporarily decreases your anxiety and doesn't affect the danger you believe you are in, you should see less and less need to engage in those rituals. Instead, your focus can be redirected towards those challenges in your life that you can do something about.

OCD Ritual Diary

Situation/time	Description of ritual	Discomfort felt %	Duration of ritual
Praying at my local church	Repeating my prayers several times	60%	15 mins
Cooking at home	Constantly checking to make sure oven is turned off	80%	Check about 15 times over 30 min period
Cleaning dishes	Washing each dish several times	70%	30 mins
Returning home	Checking several times to see if the door is locked	90%	Approximately 20 times in a two-hour period

4.10 PTSD Diary

Grey, N., Young, K. & Holmes, E. (2002). Cognitive restructuring within reliving: A treatment for peritraumatic emotional 'hotspots' in posttraumatic stress disorder. *Behavioural and Cognitive Psychotherapy*, *30*, 37–56.

Purpose

Traumatic experiences can often lead people to experience vivid and upsetting symptoms many months or years after the traumatic event. Recurring nightmares, flashbacks and intrusive images are commonplace, and can be triggered by the most banal, everyday situations. When these episodes occur, it can feel as if you are reliving the past, and your body will respond to the threat by activating the fight/flight response. If it is intense enough, you will feel as if you have no other choice but to seek to escape the situation. Unfortunately, if you do escape the situation, you reinforce the idea that you were in danger. You also teach your mind that avoidance is the best solution to your problems.

Using a PTSD Diary to record these episodes can help you understand what they are and find an alternative solution to avoidance. By putting down on paper the situation you are in and how you feel, you effectively ground yourself in the present moment and can confront your thoughts for what they are: distortions. When you stay in the situation and your anxiety reduces, it will further emphasise that your problem is not with an actual threat but with your emotional and physiological response to your anxiety. The PTSD Diary can then help you frame a more realistic assessment of the situation and come up with a new, more adaptable response.

Suitability

The PTSD Diary is for people with symptoms of PTSD. It can help with those moments where you dissociate, have flashbacks or in any other way relive your past trauma. Keep in mind that confronting trauma can be very difficult. I suggest you use the diary with the help of an experienced therapist, if at all possible.

How to use

Whenever you feel divorced from the present and experience intrusive thoughts or flashbacks, ground yourself back in the present (Grounding, Chapter 3, p.66), breathe (Square Breathing Technique, Chapter 3, p.56) and take out this diary. Record where you are, who you are with and any triggers that might have made you feel this way. Describe your emotions and your physical reactions, and then turn to your thoughts. Your thoughts might be distortions of reality – you may be perceiving a threat where there is none. If this is the case, explore this discrepancy further and record it, however unpleasant it might feel.

Ask yourself if the thoughts you are having are due to the situation you are currently in or if they are the remnants of unresolved trauma in your past. Try to judge the situation you are in without reference to the past. What do your senses tell you is real? Your instincts might tell you one thing, but what does the rational part of your brain say? Record these in the Realistic Assessment section. Finally, think of a new response that matches your more realistic assessment of the situation. If, for example, you no longer believe you are in danger, there is no reason to run away. Instead, you can redirect your attention towards what is actually happening in the here and now and free yourself from your distorted thoughts.

PTSD Diary

Situation	Emotion	Physical reaction	Distorted thoughts/ images	Realistic assessment	New response		
Walking down the street	Fear, panic	Walking faster, keeping away from strangers	I am going to get attacked. Image of a dark shadow swooping down	Nobody around me looks like a threat.	Focus on breathing, release the tension in my muscles		
Going down into the metro	Terror, confusion	Can't breathe, throat gets dry, stay away from the walls	I will be trapped. The walls are closing in on me	Many people use the metro without issue. The walls are not moving closer	Focus my attention on where I have to go and future plans		
Speaking with a friend	Nervousness, scared	Heart rate increases, start to sweat, speak less	Image of being kicked over and over again	My friend would not want to harm me. I'm safe with them	Change the subject and absorb myself in the conversation		

Chapter 5. Cognitive restructuring

Introduction

Our thoughts allow us to make sense of the world, to conceptualise what is in front of us and to extract significance from our experiences. The thoughts are not always entirely accurate, but this does not necessarily result in anything worse than a misplaced confidence in our abilities or a maintaining of biased opinions. However, when we are struggling with life problems, we are much more likely to apply unhelpful thinking styles that emphasise our perceived faults or shortcomings. We overestimate danger or fail to look at a situation from a balanced perspective. In these cases, it is not uncommon to become trapped in our own subjectivity. As our emotional state worsens, so does the nature of our thoughts, until it is difficult to see any escape. This chapter is concerned with challenging these unhelpful thoughts and thinking styles and looking for evidence that suggests that they are not true.

The chapter begins with Unhelpful Thinking Styles (p.92), which looks at naming the thinking styles that distort reality. These can then be disputed in various ways, as the chapter goes on to explore. You can look for competing evidence that reduces the likelihood that what you are saying is true, through the Thought-Disputing Model (p.94). You can look at the costs and benefits of holding a specific thought and re-evaluate whether it is worth maintaining it by using the Cost/Benefit Analysis (p.98). All these methods are concerned with challenging the premises on which your thoughts are based. If you can start to perceive other ways of framing your problems, you can begin to see a way out of your current predicament.

Many of the models in this chapter recognise that challenging your beliefs requires being able to identify the right tools for the job. Worry Tree (p.100) uses a familiar flowchart diagram to help you work out how to deal with different types of worries. Similarly, the Theory A/B Model (p.102) suggests you see your problem as either a practical problem requiring problem-solving skills or a problem of perception. How you proceed depends on which theory sounds most accurate to you.

In some situations, you will find that thought challenging is not enough on its own to see steady progress. This can sometimes be attributed to core beliefs and rules about yourself, others and the world that are at odds with reality. These beliefs are deep seated and develop slowly over a lifetime, so they are much more resistant to change. Nevertheless, recognising them and the dysfunctional role they play in your life is the first step towards change. The second half of this chapter is dedicated to exploring and challenging them.

Some of the formulations in Chapter 1 may have helped you identify any unhealthy core beliefs you may hold. Consider using the material in this chapter to understand your history with them, and how to best put them into words. As with your thoughts, consider the evidence you might have for holding these beliefs. Often, they originate in childhood experiences or in particularly traumatic experiences that were left unresolved. In many cases, this evidence is far outweighed by more recent events that contradict your beliefs, but you have, for one reason or another, neglected them and held onto your original experiences. Core Belief Challenging (p.106) and the Evidence Table for Core Beliefs (p.108) both provide space for you to consider how valid your underlying beliefs are.

Core beliefs often shape our behaviour. If we believe that such and such is true, we will create rules that govern how we should act in certain circumstances. It is these inflexible rules that often cause friction with others and highlight that change is needed. A model such as Cycle of Beliefs, Rules and Behaviours (p.110) clarifies how this process works and how it can be maintained for many years. Hopefully, at the same time, it shows that if you modify some of your thoughts and behaviours or change your rules into values (using the Rules into Values model, p.112), you can target these stubborn core beliefs and make gradual progress towards your goals.

5.1 Unhelpful Thinking Styles

Beck, A.T. (1976). *Cognitive therapy and the emotional disorders.* International Universities Press.

Purpose

The purpose of Unhelpful Thinking Styles is to help us recognise our mistakes and errors of judgement. By identifying those styles that distort our thinking process, we can reduce or stop them from affecting our mood. Doing so should better equip us to handle challenges that are created not from reality but from our take on reality. This subtle difference can have a profound impact on whether we allow anger, fear or sadness to overwhelm us or if, by taking a different interpretation, we can reach a more compassionate and generous space from which to reach out to others.

Suitability

No one is entirely free from thinking in ways that misrepresent reality. Unhelpful Thinking Styles is designed for people who find themselves falling into the same counterproductive thinking styles time and time again. It can be of particular use to those who are feeling quite low and have started to view the world in a negative light. Simply naming these cognitive traps can do much to lessen their hold on you, but if that is not enough, I recommend you pair this worksheet with the Thought-Disputing Model (p.94).

How to use

Start by reading the thinking styles listed below and ask yourself if you have used any of them recently. Next, turn to the worksheet and write down the situations and your thoughts and emotions when using those particular styles. If more than one example comes to mind, use another sheet of paper to write them down. If there are some styles that you don't recognise in yourself, leave them empty.

- **Tunnel vision/mental filter** – Deciding to look at a situation from one perspective while ignoring other ways of viewing it.
- **Jumping to conclusions** – Imagining that, because a certain thing happened, a particular something else will follow straight after.
- **Personalising** – Taking offence at others' actions, even though there is little or no evidence that their actions were directed towards you.
- **Catastrophising** – Picturing the very worst-case scenarios happening to you or those around you.
- **Black-and-white thinking** – Seeing the world from an either/or perspective. Ignoring the complexity of an issue.
- **Should/must thinking** – Believing that everything should or must be a certain way.
- **Over-generalising** – Applying one specific outcome from the past to all future imagined outcomes.
- **Labelling** – Attributing to yourself or others unnecessary names that aren't deserved.
- **Emotional reasoning** – Allowing your emotions to dictate the judgements you make.
- **Magnification or/and minimisation** – Blowing small things out of proportion or failing to acknowledge the significance of things.

Unhelpful Thinking Styles

Situation	Thought	Emotions	My unhelpful thinking styles
Being praised for my performance in a play	Nobody complimented me on an aspect of my performance	I feel unrecognised, ignored	Tunnel vision/mental filter
Finding a stray hair on my partner's shoulder	My partner is cheating on me	Jealousy, betrayal	Jumping to conclusions
My team did not win first place	It was me that held the team back	I feel ashamed, disappointed in myself	Personalising
I am 5 minutes late for my interview	Everything from this point will be a disaster	Tearful, nervous, anxious	Catastrophising
Getting into an argument with my partner	Our relationship is a failure as we argue	Angry, frustrated	Black-and-white thinking
Failing to reach all my weekly targets	I should be able to hit all my weekly targets every week	Depressed, let down	Should/must thinking
Not able to put together flat-pack furniture	I am useless at everything	Distressed, sad	Overgeneralising
Too tired to do my chores today	I'm a lazy person	Exhausted, distraught	Labelling
I feel low because of the weather	The weather is going to ensure that this day is terrible	Defeated, fatalistic	Emotional reasoning
Winning an award	I was just lucky	Guilty	Magnification or/and minimisation

5.2 Thought-Disputing Model

Beck, A.T. & Beck, J.S. (1995). *Cognitive therapy: Basics and beyond*. Guilford Press.

Purpose

Sometimes it's necessary to look at our thoughts and question whether they stand up to close scrutiny. When we are feeling low or very anxious, our emotions colour the way we perceive the world. When we are already struggling to cope with life's demands, we are much more likely to expect ourselves to fail, judge ourselves harshly or find fault in others. Nevertheless, it doesn't have to be this way. It is possible to break the hold that our overly negative thoughts have on us.

The Thought-Disputing Model provides a way to look at our thoughts as another person might, with a little more objectivity and less emotional reasoning. By identifying any unhelpful thinking styles and looking for evidence for and against our thoughts, we can come to a more balanced way of looking at our situation. Perspective is not something that always comes easily, which is why this model might be helpful at times when our mental resources are limited.

Suitability

When we overly focus on the negative in our lives, our thoughts become imbalanced. We apply unhelpful thinking styles that highlight only one side of the argument. The Thought-Disputing Model is a way to realign our thinking so we can see both sides. The aim is not to eradicate the negative thoughts but rather to see the issue in a more objective manner, in the hope that this will reduce the intensity of our feelings. It is suitable for most people, but those experiencing depression or low mood might find it particularly useful.

How to use

Begin by naming a recent 'hot thought'. A hot thought is an intense thought that comes to mind immediately when you are faced with a problem or stressful situation. It is often recurring and not bound to one specific situation. Moreover, its emotional intensity is often derived from the significance that you give it. Many hot thoughts have to do with your idea of self, the world and your performance. When recording your hot thought, it can help to write it as a complete sentence that starts with 'I…' This can ground the thought in your lived experience and ensure that it doesn't become too abstract. Once you have a specific hot thought, rate your belief in it on a scale of 0–100.

Now ask yourself if this hot thought falls victim to any unhelpful thinking styles. Use the Unhelpful Thinking Styles worksheet (p.92) to remind yourself of these and to check if you are using any. You can highlight several styles or leave the space blank if none come to mind. Move on to listing all the evidence you have that supports your hot thought. Try not to include opinions or superstitions or any other factually questionable beliefs. Follow this by listing all the evidence you have against your hot thought. This might be more challenging, especially if the hot thought is something you have carried with you for many years. It can help here to draw on personal experience of past achievements that contradict the hot thought.

Finally, take a step back and look at what you have written. Does the accumulation of competing evidence against your hot thought and the recognition of unhelpful thinking styles transform that initial thought in any way? If so, rewrite your hot thought in a way that highlights this new-found balance. Look at the score you gave your belief in the hot thought at the start of this exercise and re-score it. Has the score reduced at all?

Cognitive restructuring

Thought-Disputing Model

Hot thought

I am a heartless person

70 %

Unhelpful thinking style

Labelling

Black-and-white thinking

Mental filter

Evidence for...	Evidence against...
I didn't help my friend when she needed me	I often give gifts and tokens of kindness to friends and family
I don't get upset when others are in tears	I often ruminate and obsess about others' reactions
My mother tells me that I am a cold person	I used to volunteer for a local charity
	I am polite to strangers

Balanced thought

There are some instances where I struggle to show the appropriate emotional reaction and spend the time helping those close to me. On the whole, though, there are many appreciative things that I do that show I have love and care for others

90 %

5.3 Decatastrophising Model

Ellis, A. (1962). *Reason and emotion in psychotherapy*. Lyle Stuart.

Purpose

To catastrophise is to see a situation as much worse than it actually is. The smallest obstacle seems like an overwhelming challenge. When you catastrophise, your mind can feel as if it is in overdrive, running through a thousand scenarios, each worse than the last. This can reduce your motivation to do anything. After all, if you think all your efforts will end in disaster, why bother in the first place? Unfortunately this means that you never test those thoughts against reality. If you did, most likely you would discover that the only obstacle was your catastrophising.

The Decatastrophising Model can be used to question these thoughts and test if they have any basis in reality. By searching for evidence and imagining the long-term consequences of your worries coming true, you may be able to view them in a more accepting and tolerant way. They will not have the same emotional strength as before and you will be less inclined to see them as debilitating. This can free you to act, unfettered by unrealistic fears.

Suitability

This is a useful model for people with anxiety who find themselves frequently fearing the worst. Using the Decatastrophising Model can help you test out whether your worries are backed up by evidence and/or if there is a more reasonable forecast of what might occur in the future. By asking you to record how you might feel in the future if the worry came true, it can reveal your resilience, help you put the worry into perspective and encourage tolerance of things that are outside your control.

How to use

Start by highlighting a recent catastrophic worry. Be specific and present it as a clear statement. Now write down all the evidence you have that it will come true. Try to avoid emotional judgements or assumptions about how the world works. Be wary of over-generalising and assuming that, because something happened in the past, it will certainly happen again. Test out that what you are writing down is evidence – can you imagine anyone arguing against it? If not, it's likely to have truth.

Now ask yourself what is the worst that could happen if your catastrophic thought were to come true. Make sure you only look at the direct consequences of the worry happening. If you miss your interview, for example, you might not get the job. This would be a direct consequence. Try to avoid allowing that thought to snowball and become, 'If I don't get the job, I won't be able to pay my bills and I'll lose my home and my whole life will collapse.' It's very easy for catastrophic worries to become unmanageable in this way. After you have written the worst-case scenario, move on to the best. If the worry does come true, how could things still turn out alright? Recording this can disarm worries of a lot of their power – it suggests that, even if the feared outcome were to occur, you might still be able to cope with it.

The last section invites you to imagine how you would feel if the original worry did come true – not how you'd feel in the moment but in one week, one month and one year in the future. This again can reduce the significance and emotional impact of the worry. You might feel really bad if your fears came true, but would you still feel the same, or even remember the worry, one year down the line? Time can be a great healer. Allow yourself the luxury of imagining a future where your worries have come true but you are able to shrug them off and continue with your journey.

Decatastrophising Model

What is the catastrophic worry?

That my child will be in danger if I let him out of my sight

What evidence suggests that it might come true?

He is always getting into trouble when my back is turned

He hurt himself falling off a swing two years ago

I read in the news of all these terrible things happening in my neighbourhood

There are cars in the street outside that speed by very fast

My friend's child had to go to A&E because he burned himself on the stove when he was left unsupervised in the kitchen

What is the worst that could happen?

My child might end up in hospital

What is the best-case scenario?

That my child will learn on his own to be careful

If the worry does come true, what are the chances you'll be okay in...		
One week _10_ %	One month _30_ %	One year _80_ %

5.4 Cost/Benefit Analysis

Ellis, A. & Dryden, W. (1997). *The practice of rational-emotive behavior therapy*. Springer.

Purpose

We have all done a pros-and-cons list at some point in our life. By comparing the downsides and upsides of a specific choice, we can feel more confident that the choice we are making will better align with our goals. When we are struggling, we adopt many unhealthy coping strategies and unhelpful thinking styles. These can be increasingly resistant to change, especially if we start to feel progressively worse. A Cost/Benefit Analysis allows us to re-examine these thoughts and behaviours and explore what the consequences would be if we changed them.

It can be very motivating to see what we might gain from making a change to our life, but it also can be quite scary to recognise the cost as well. Few choices are all benefit with no cost, and those that are rarely need to be analysed and understood at a deeper level. Use this worksheet to better understand the significance of what change means for you. Ultimately, the solution you decide to implement should acknowledge the costs while emphasising the benefits. Doing so can help you see more clearly what you have to gain by making a change in your life.

Suitability

In our head, we usually weigh up the pros and cons of acting or thinking a certain way. When that isn't sufficient, a cost/benefit analysis can help us come up with an adaptive solution that recognises the costs of acting a certain way but also highlights what can be gained if we change our behaviour or thoughts. This model is suitable for anyone who is contemplating a change in either their behaviour or their way of seeing the world and themselves.

How to use

Start by selecting a behaviour or thought that might be holding you back in some way and that you wish to change. You might want to choose a behaviour that is putting you in conflict with others or one that is causing you distress and affecting your mental wellbeing. Or you might want to choose a self-limiting thought or a way of perceiving reality that is at odds with your values. Provided that you are open to the idea of change, most thoughts or behaviours can be suitable.

Move on to list all the costs of that change. What will you lose if you make a change? How could change result in your circumstances becoming more difficult? Score each of these costs on a scale of 1–10 where 10 suggests that the particular cost is of the utmost importance to you and 1 suggests you would barely notice any negative consequences. Now repeat the process for benefits. Try to imagine what the benefits would be if you were able to carry through the change you have in mind, and score them as to their relative importance to you.

The last step is to take all the costs and benefits and strike a compromise. Ignoring all the costs of a change might very well sabotage your efforts. So imagine an adaptive solution that brings the high-scoring benefits but makes room for and acknowledges the costs that the change will entail. In practical terms, this can mean that your change might take a slightly different form to the one you first imagined. Hopefully, this new form will seem more easily implemented than previous more radical solutions.

Cognitive restructuring

Cost/Benefit Analysis

Thought/behaviour to be changed

Stop isolating myself in my room when I feel low

Costs	1–10
I will no longer have a safe refuge from others	7
I will have to hide my emotions better in front of others	6
There will be nowhere that I can be alone with my thoughts	3

Benefits	1-10
I will be more productive during the day	8
I might get along better with people if I don't close down and hide away	7
I won't feel as depressed	10
I won't get trapped in the negative spiral of self-critical thoughts	6
I might learn to deal with my problems when they arise	5

Adaptive solution

I will try to monitor my emotions better and exchange my isolation for activities that can reduce the pressure I feel. I will try to make these social and not be afraid of showing negative emotions if those feelings arise. If I need to be alone, I will try not to allow myself to ruminate about past events but use the time to think of productive things I can do with my time in the coming week.

5.5 Worry Tree

Butler, G. & Hope, T. (2007). *Manage your mind: The mental fitness guide*. Oxford University Press.

Purpose

Worries come in all shapes and sizes. There are many different ways to categorise them, but one of the most effective is by the degree of power you have to resolve them. Some worries you can do something about straight away. Others you will need to plan to deal with in the future, and some worries are too hypothetical for any practical solution to help. Worry Tree is a flow diagram that can help you distinguish between these three types of worry. The idea is that, if you know what type of worry you are dealing with, you can craft an appropriate solution for it. As such, this diagram serves to help you recognise the options you have available to resolve your worries before they become overwhelming.

Suitability

Worry Tree is helpful for anyone experiencing anxiety. Identifying and separating your worries into three categories can make it easier to address how you will tackle them. The model works well with a number of other models, such as Stress Quadrant (Chapter 2, p.40) and Worry Time (Chapter 6, p.120) and any of the relaxation techniques in Chapter 3. I suggest you use this model as a gateway to other models in this book and as a guide to when best to use them.

How to use

Start at the foot of the tree by writing down one specific worry that has been playing on your mind recently. Next, follow the arrows and answer whether your worry is something that you can't do anything about, can't do anything about right now, or can do something about right now. If the worry is outside your control, make the decision to redirect your attention elsewhere, using the redirection techniques in Chapter 3. This might be towards a mundane activity or an activity that gives you pleasure. If the anxiety is intense, you might want to redirect your attention towards your breathing until you are calmer.

If your worry is something within your control but can't be dealt with immediately, consider the resources you have at your disposal. Can you schedule a time in the future to deal with the issue? Think about what therapeutic or non-therapeutic tools might help you with this.

Finally, if your worry is about something that you can solve right now, act on this. Either in your mind or on paper, note some solutions that you can put into place right now. If you are faced with some tough choices, consider using the Cost/Benefit Analysis worksheet (p.98) to problem-solve them. Then act on your decision.

If you use this model several times, you will start to collect a number of solutions and techniques to help you with each type of worry. It can be a good idea to record them on the worksheets so that, when faced with further challenges, you can reflect on what has worked for you in the past.

Cognitive restructuring 101

Worry Tree

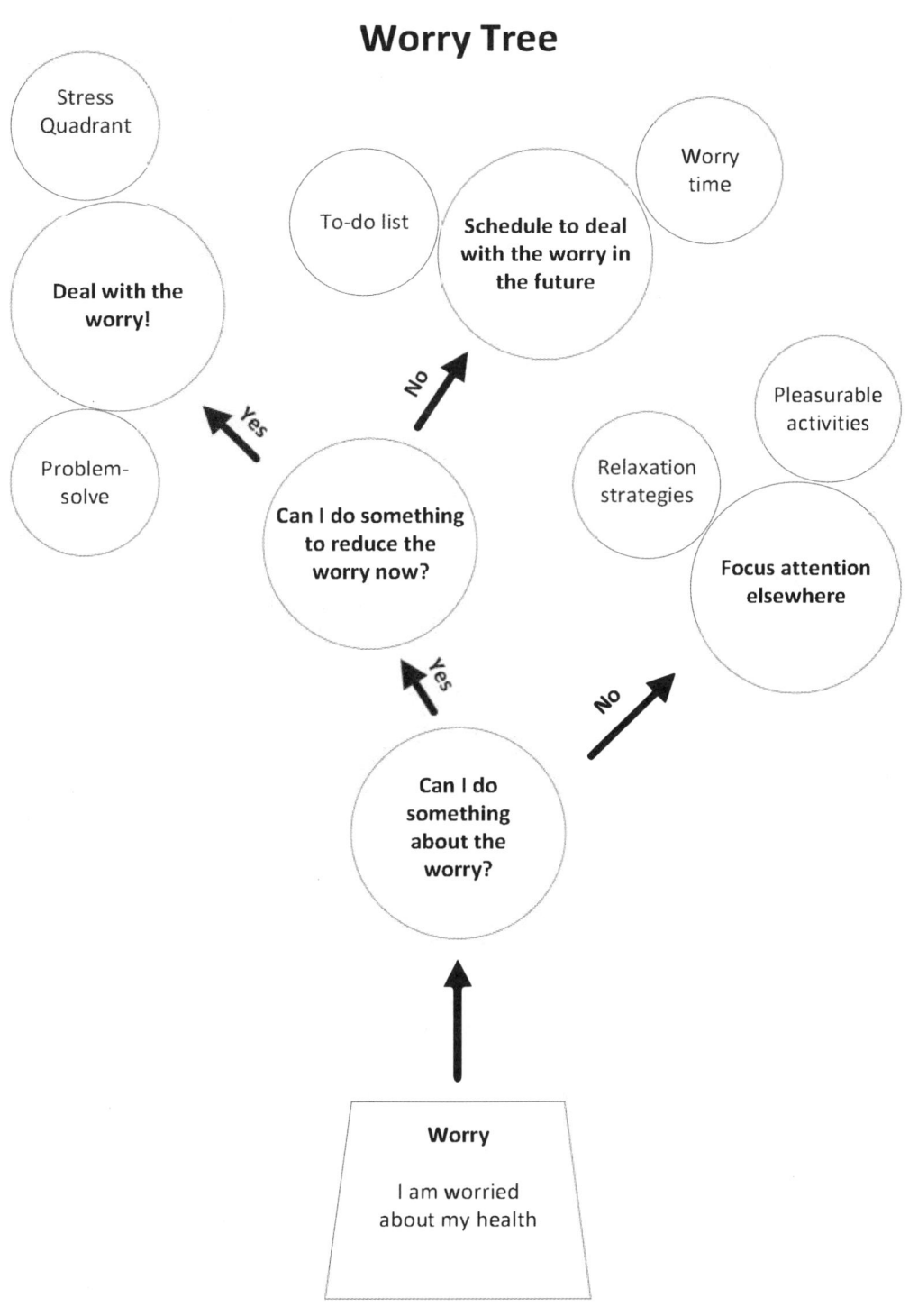

5.6 Theory A/B Model

Wells, A. (1997). *Cognitive therapy of anxiety disorders: A practice manual and conceptual guide*. John Wiley & Sons.

Purpose

Often, when we decide that change is necessary, we have come to this conclusion because of the difficulties in our lives. It is these difficulties that we want resolved. Whether it's poor sleep, panic attacks, lack of motivation or low energy, we want an immediate solution that removes the symptoms. After some reflection, though, we may realise the true problem is our way of looking at the world and ourselves. In that case, to treat the symptoms and to ignore the cause of the problem will lead only to short-lived, superficial change.

The Theory A/B Model is designed to highlight how we all have an underlying theory for what is maintaining our problems. This is Theory A. As with all theories, there will be some evidence to support it and there will be certain consequences of believing it. Some of those consequences will be the negative symptoms that are causing you so much difficulty in your life. It is possible that, by adopting another view on why you feel the way you do, Theory B, you will understand that your difficulties are maintained by your current underlying beliefs, and that, if they are changed, your problems will change too.

Suitability

People who have difficulty seeing alternative explanations for their problems might find the Theory A/B Model helpful. By proposing an alternative theory for your problem, it can help you question the underlying beliefs that might be maintaining it. The comparison should make clear that how you frame a problem can contribute to maintaining it or allow you to resolve it. The model has particular resonance for people with OCD, health/social anxiety and panic disorder. It is only suitable for use with problems with a strong psychological component, not issues of practical day-to-day living.

How to use

Begin by stating your problem under Theory A. Make sure that you only state one problem per worksheet and that you use clear, straightforward language. Be sure to state a belief or something that you believe to be a fact. Avoid listing the symptoms of your problem. Theory A/B Model will only work with those problems that have a strong psychological component. Practical issues such as housing, domestic abuse or drug addiction are all valid problems, but they require far more than a change in mindset to resolve them, which is what this model is designed to explore.

On the other side of the worksheet, under Theory B, rewrite the problem as a belief, an unhelpful thinking style or in any way that emphasises how the problem might be one of perception and not reality. Then look for hard evidence that suggests either theory is true. You will most likely come up with evidence for both columns. Write whatever comes to mind, but once you have completed the worksheet, return to this stage and reflect on the validity of the evidence given here. How much might be the result of overgeneralising or lack of context? You can use the Thought-Disputing Model (p.94) here if you think it might help produce more balanced thoughts.

At the bottom of the model, explore what you would need to do if either theory were true. This is intended to highlight the coping techniques you are already using and the techniques you could be using if you were to regard your problem as a psychological issue. The contrast should be quite distinct. Hopefully the techniques in the second column should seem easier to apply than those in the first.

Theory A/B Model

Theory A

The problem is...

I am a fraud

What is the hard evidence that this is true?

People don't know everything about me

I have secrets that I haven't disclosed to those close to me

I have lied on my CV

I made up things in conversations about myself

What do I need to do if theory A is true?

Stay on guard

Monitor my emotions and behaviours to make sure I don't do anything that will expose me

Over-analyse situations to make sure I haven't come across wrong

Theory B

The problem is self-doubt, worry, rumination that...

I believe I am a fraud and I worry that people might find out

What is the hard evidence that this is true?

I spend hours thinking about what others think of me

I ask friends for reassurance

I avoid situations that might expose the truth about me

I can't sleep because of the worry

What do I need to do if theory B is true?

Focus on facts, not subjective feelings

Accept that I can't be in control of everything

Replace worry with problem-solving

Stay in the present

5.7 Health Anxiety Change Model

Furer, P., Walker, J.R. & Stein, M.B. (2007). *Treating health anxiety and fear of death: A practitioner's guide.* Springer.

Purpose

Health anxiety is excessive worrying about your health and an over-reliance on checking and reassurance behaviour to reduce those worries. The key to understanding this condition is in the words 'excessive' and 'over-reliance'. It is normal for people to want to identify any negative physical symptoms that they feel, perhaps by searching the internet for a cause or asking their doctor. If these attempts have always come back with no firm answers and the symptoms can be explained as side effects of anxiety, this could be an indication that the source of your problems is in your mind, not your body.

So how do you resolve these worries and unhelpful behaviours? The Health Anxiety Change Model illustrates how your worries are triggered by specific situations and then amplified by the very behaviours you imagine are helping you solve those worries. By reflecting on this situation and analysing how certain unhelpful thinking styles increase your worries and make them overwhelming, you can propose alternative ways of looking at your situation that minimise the possibility of your health being at actual risk. Instead of checking with more doctors or searching for more information online, you make room for the idea that you need to change your perception that you are constantly in danger if you are to resolve your anxieties.

Suitability

The Health Anxiety Change Model can be useful in understanding how a specific situational trigger leads to health worries, checking behaviour and unhelpful thinking styles. It also allows you to evaluate how effective your current strategies are and, if necessary, find alternative explanations that might better fit the description of what you are experiencing. While you are doing this, the model reminds you why you are challenging your beliefs – essentially, in order to reach your goals and values. If you feel your motivation dwindling, remember how important those goals and values are to you and how you will feel once they've been accomplished. You should use this model only if you have some insight into your health anxiety and recognise it as playing a significant part in your difficulties.

How to use

Begin the first part of the worksheet by listing a recent specific situation that caused negative emotions, health worries and some form of checking/reassurance behaviour. Once you have recorded this, ask yourself if any of the unhelpful thinking styles listed in the worksheet might have something to do with your health anxiety. Circle any that do.

Then turn to your behaviour. How effective is the checking/reassurance behaviour that you act out? Does the relief that it offers last long? Or does the anxiety return quite soon after and you end up repeating similar thoughts and behaviours? If you feel that you want to experiment and try alternative behaviour and thinking styles, write down what these might look like. Include anything that you have learned in this book about anxiety and maintenance cycles.

Now make room in your mind for the possibility that your current behaviour has actually been maintaining your problems and not helping you at all. This can be quite difficult as it might interfere with other core beliefs. Try to entertain the possibility by reminding yourself how important change is to your goals and values. The methods that you have been trying for so long have probably moved you away from these goals, so perhaps it is time to try something different.

Health Anxiety Change Model

Trigger
Noting a pain in my chest

Initial emotional reaction
Puzzlement, discomfort, fear

Health worry
Is this another complication following the surgery that I had a year ago?

Checking/reassurance behaviour
Monitoring my heart rate and blood pressure

Booking an appointment with the GP

- Catastrophizing
- Uncertainty avoidance
- Negative filter

Fatalistic thinking   Thought-action fusion

How effective is checking behaviour?
My heart rate was quite high, but that could have been because I was getting quite anxious thinking about everything. My blood pressure was normal, but I'm not sure how accurate my device is. It made me want to speak to a doctor, even though in the past my GP has not been very helpful

Values and goals
This will move me closer to my goals as if I don't have any worries about my physical health, I can resume those daily activities that I have stopped

Making room
I will need to make room for the possibility that a lot of my symptoms could be associated with anxiety and there is no significant underlying health condition

Alternative response
To refocus my attention away from my body

To practise visual imagery

5.8 Core Belief Challenging

Wenzel, A. (2012). Modification of core beliefs in cognitive therapy. In I. Reis De Oliveira (Ed.), *Cognitive-behavioral therapy* (pp.17–34). InTech.

Purpose

Once you understand which of your core beliefs are impacting your health negatively, you may wish to challenge and revise them. Core Belief Challenging can help you face these destructive beliefs and test whether there really is enough evidence to believe in them. Often, once you untangle your unhelpful thinking styles and faulty assumptions, you can see that there is little rationale for holding these beliefs. This realisation can help you create a more balanced belief that acknowledges your emotional reasoning but doesn't let it overwhelm all the opposing evidence that points in a different direction.

Suitability

When you have identified unhealthy core beliefs, the next stage is to challenge those beliefs and question how much evidence there is for believing them. Core Belief Challenging can help you see how much evidence there is that your core belief is unsubstantiated. The creation of more balanced core beliefs can help many people, but this worksheet should only be used by those who believe their core beliefs are responsible for their problems and when other methods, such as relaxation techniques and behavioural activation, have been unsuccessful.

How to use

Start by recording on the worksheet the unhealthy core belief that you wish to challenge. This belief might involve unrealistic expectations, poor self-image or overly pessimistic forecasts for the future. Remember that a core belief is a deeply entrenched belief that affects how you see the world and will frequently impact the quality of your life.

Next, write down what evidence you have for believing that your core belief might be an inaccurate representation of reality. Do certain life experiences contradict it? Can testimonials of friends or family provide arguments against it? It can sometimes be difficult to think of compelling evidence for why your core beliefs might not be true. If you are finding this is the case, consider asking your therapist or a close friend to help. The perspective of another person can highlight those pieces of evidence that you might not be able to see.

When you have collected enough evidence, use it to create a balanced core belief that is more compassionate to yourself and less black and white. These balanced beliefs should not be an explicit refutation of your previous unhealthy core beliefs. Rather, they should be a gentle rewording that allows you to see how inflexible your previous thinking was and the benefits change could bring.

Core Belief Challenging

Core belief to be challenged

I am not likeable

Experiences that challenge core belief

I have a very good, childhood friend

People occasionally ask me to do them favours

My dog enjoys my company

When I was younger I had a few good friends/classmates

When I left my last job I got a 'wish you well' card from all my colleagues

Sometimes my stories/jokes make people laugh

I am very polite and never get angry with others

I was able to socialise at my work Christmas party

Balanced core belief

There are some situations and instances where I can see that I am liked, only those situations are few and far between. A lot of my evidence centres around work, perhaps because I do so little socialising outside work. I find this quite difficult as it is really hard to get in others' heads to figure out if they like me or not. I guess I'm trying to mind-read a lot, where instead I should be focusing on the evidence in front of me and increasing my opportunities to interact with others.

5.9 Evidence Table for Core Beliefs

Riso, L.P., du Toit, P.L., Stein, D.J. & Young, J.E. (Eds.) (2007). *Cognitive schemas and core beliefs in psychological problems: A scientist-practitioner guide.* American Psychological Association.

Purpose

A table is made steady by its legs. Too few legs and it will fall over. Our beliefs operate in a similar fashion. If our beliefs do not stand on solid foundations, they are likely to be superseded by new beliefs that are better able to explain reality. So it is with our core beliefs, except because they are so deeply entrenched in how we see ourselves, others and the world, they are much tougher to change, despite all the evidence that might be against them. Occasionally these core beliefs can clash and contradict each other, resulting in a great deal of mental anguish as we are unable to resolve them in a way that allows us to properly function in society. To avoid this discomfort, we hold firmly to our initial core beliefs and refuse to accept contrary beliefs that might destabilise our sense of self.

The Evidence Table for Core Beliefs allows you to examine any unhealthy core beliefs you might hold and the evidence that supports them. Often stating the evidence for an unhealthy core belief can make you see how weak or scant that evidence is and how your life might change if you adopt a more balanced alternative.

Suitability

Unhealthy core beliefs do not come out of nowhere. They are often the product of unpleasant life experiences and are maintained by our desire not to have those experiences repeated. Understanding the evidence that supports our unhealthy core beliefs allows us to better challenge the beliefs that they support. The Evidence Table for Core Beliefs is suitable for people looking to explore the basis of their core beliefs and contrast them with healthier alternatives that might provide relief from their difficulties. But to even anticipate changing a core belief requires that you are in the right headspace and open to change. You need to prepare yourself accordingly before you use this model.

How to use

On the first table in the worksheet, write down the unhealthy core belief that you want to challenge. Now turn the worksheet on one side and address each of the table's legs. Each leg represents a supporting belief, memory or piece of evidence that explains why you hold this unhealthy core belief in the first place and, more importantly, why you hold onto it to this day. When the worksheet uses the term 'evidence', it means it in the loosest sense of the word. Almost anything that you believe to be evidence qualifies, as it is the significance that you give to it that matters, not whether it will pass any objective standard. Nevertheless, if you feel the evidence you record on the legs of the table is particularly flawed, it is certainly worth asking yourself if you are applying any unhelpful thinking styles that might be responsible for distorting your sense of self, others and the world.

Once you have completed the first table, move on to the second. This table should be used to create a healthy core belief that involves the same issues as your unhealthy core belief but is far more balanced and generous with its understanding of reality. After you have written down this healthier core belief, add reasons why it might be a clearer, more accurate way of perceiving the world. If you compare the evidence with that in the first table, hopefully you should see that it looks far more plausible than the evidence used to support your unhealthy core belief. If you run out of table legs and have more accumulating evidence, feel free to add further legs to stabilise your healthy core belief still further.

Evidence Table for Core Beliefs

Unhealthy core belief

I always make mistakes

- When I made a driving error last week, the cars behind me started honking
- My partner criticises the way I dress
- I recently learned I was pronouncing a word wrong. When I was corrected, people laughed
- I was yelled at as a child for making mistakes in class
- My parents used to criticise me for not doing as well as my brother

Healthy core belief

Mistakes happen, and though sometimes embarrassing, usually have little negative consequence

- I have never knowingly failed a job interview because of my choice of tie
- My partner often has trouble with maths, but she is able to shrug off mistakes
- When I make small driving errors, I don't get a ticket or lose my licence
- I see others laugh off their mistakes and weaknesses and make a joke of them
- I sometimes make accounting mistakes and when I confess to them it is acknowledged and we move on to the next point

5.10 Cycle of Beliefs, Rules and Behaviours

Beck, A.T., & Beck, J.S. (1995). *Cognitive therapy: Basics and beyond*. Guilford Press.

Purpose

When you begin to explore your thinking processes, I suggest you begin with those thoughts that arise in distressing situations. These automatic thoughts can be understood in the context of the situation and can be connected with your physical symptoms, emotions and behaviours. While they can be dealt with in the moment, occasionally they persist, and underlying beliefs about yourself, others and the world become apparent. These core beliefs influence how you see the world and will lead to rules and assumptions based on them. The problems arise when you hold unhealthy core beliefs that are unwarranted and for which you have little evidence. Consequently, the rules you form and the behaviours you enact to keep them in place will lead to counterproductive outcomes, based as they are on faulty premises.

It is for this reason that some behaviours are so difficult to change. You are not simply changing what you do; you are changing the rules that govern your actions and the underlying beliefs that are at the centre of who you are as a person. Cycle of Beliefs, Rules and Behaviours highlights this complexity and can point you in the direction of meaningful change.

Suitability

Our unhealthy core beliefs are not maintained through stubbornness and perseverance but by the rules we hold and the behaviours that follow from them. If we wish to dismantle these beliefs, we need to understand how our rules and behaviours prevent us from ever challenging them. This worksheet should be completed only after you have identified your unhealthy core beliefs. Provided you have done so, Cycle of Beliefs, Rules and Behaviours is suitable for anyone who recognises the limitations of their beliefs and has managed to see how they are holding them back from growth.

How to use

Begin by writing down on the worksheet the unhealthy core belief that you wish to explore. This should be stated in clear, unambiguous terms. Follow this by writing down the rules that follow from this core belief. For example, if you believe that everything important in your life is outside your control, a rule might be, 'If something bad happens to me, then I can't be held responsible for it,' or 'If I fail at something, then there is no point in me trying again.' As you can see, these rules often take an 'If… then…' structure. As these rules and assumptions about how things work are so closely tied to your core beliefs, it is very difficult to change one rule without changing the whole superstructure around it.

Once you have identified these rules, try to recall the critical incident that might have created them. This can often be something quite far in the past – a one-off event or a prolonged experience in childhood. Alternatively, it can be a more recent traumatic event that acted as a catalyst and awoke these beliefs within you. It is important at this stage to ask how your behaviours keep your unhealthy core belief in place. How do they prevent you from seeing how disconnected they are from reality? Often these behaviours can involve avoidance or reassurance, which might temporarily reduce your distress while simultaneously maintaining your belief in the validity of your core belief. It is this crucial question that the worksheet aims to help you answer. How does your cycle of beliefs, rules and behaviours maintain itself? Once you understand how this cycle operates, you can begin to take it apart and free yourself from its tyranny.

Cycle of Beliefs, Rules and Behaviours

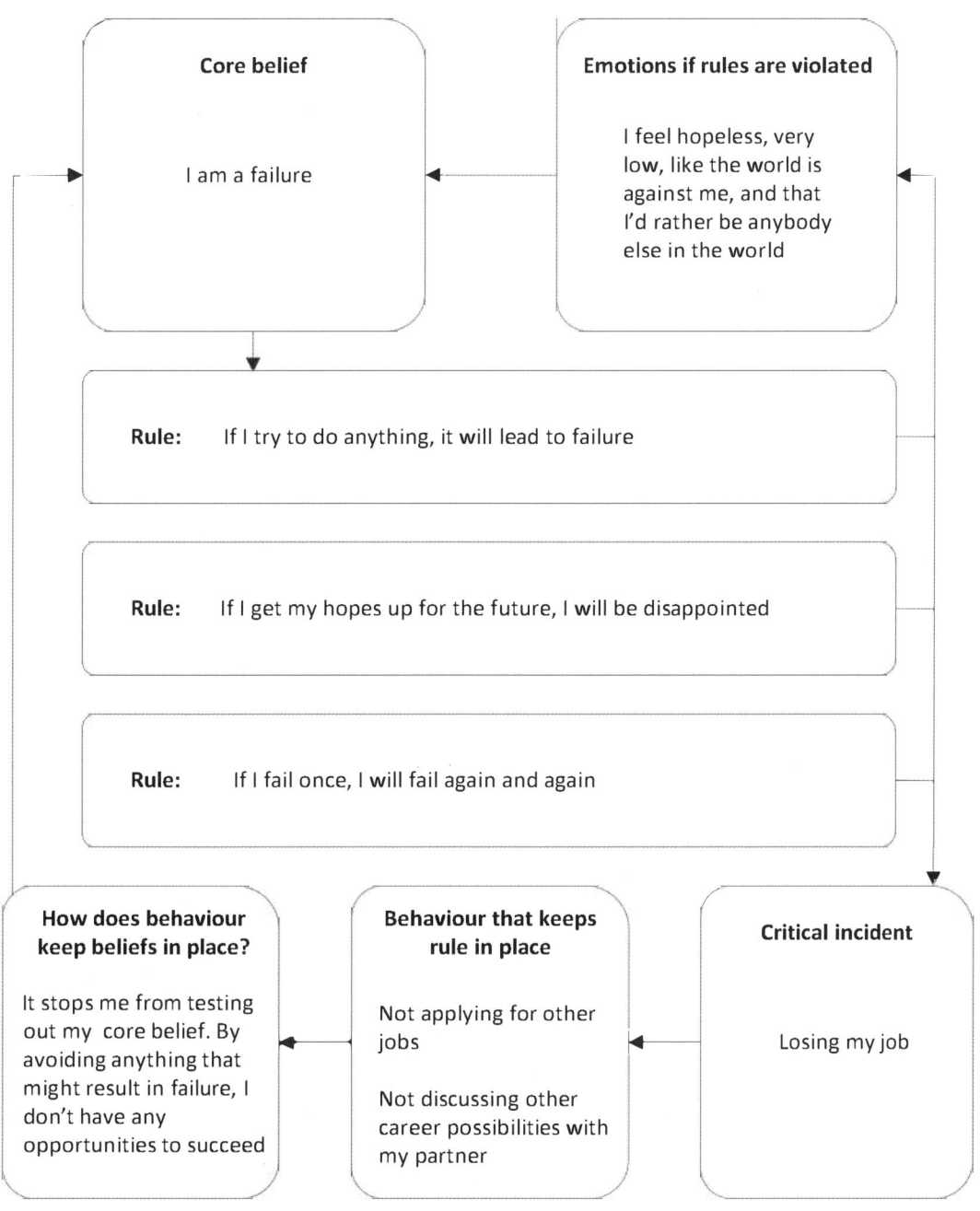

5.11 Rules into Values

Wilson, K.G. & Murrell, A.R. (2004). Values work in acceptance and commitment therapy: Setting a course for behavioral treatment. In S.C. Hayes, V.M. Follette & M. Linehan (Eds.), *Mindfulness and acceptance: Expanding the cognitive-behavioral tradition* (pp.120–151). Guilford Press.

Purpose

We all hold core beliefs about ourselves and the world. These beliefs influence how we engage with others and impact our sense of identity. We create rules founded on these beliefs that tell us how to act, how to respond to others and how to deal with threats. Occasionally these rules are counterproductive and lead to outcomes that are not aligned with our goals. Nevertheless, we hold onto them because they support our values and our underlying beliefs about how the world works.

While it is possible to change your core beliefs directly, it is also worth looking at your rules and questioning if there are alternative ways of applying them. Rules into Values helps you search for the underlying values that uphold your rules. By accepting these values but examining whether your rules can be made more flexible, you can gently challenge the way you see the world and your place in it.

Suitability

Rules into Values is a helpful model if you want to explore how certain rules might limit your growth and result in unhelpful outcomes. It does so not by rejecting the rules outright but by identifying the values that lie behind them. As such, this model can be paired well with Exploring Values (Chapter 2, p.50), as a better understanding of where your values originate can help you change your rules and make them more flexible. Other models in this chapter that involve core beliefs can also complement Rules into Values and should be used to further any insights gathered here.

How to use

On the far left of the worksheet, begin by listing the personal rules you have created that are self-limiting. These rules can be framed as 'I must...' or 'I should...' They can also be structured as 'If so, ...' and 'So, if true, then I need to...' What makes a rule self-limiting is if it hinders you from expressing yourself fully or if it interferes with your goals or contradicts certain values. Rules are often framed as either/or and are resistant to nuance or complexity. Once you have identified these rules, ask yourself what the unhelpful outcomes of applying them are, and write that down. These usually involve your behaviour or distressful situations that you find yourself in because of your actions.

Next, take these rules and examine the values that underpin them: write on the worksheet the personal values behind your rules. A value is an aspirational target that you can direct your life towards. For instance, if your self-limiting rule is that you must never fail, the value behind that might be that you want to succeed in life. There is nothing wrong with holding that value. It is only when it begins to be applied inflexibly to everything you do that it becomes unsupportable. Imagine how you could hold onto your values, but at the same time apply modified versions of your rules that are more generous and forgiving to yourself. Use the last box in the model to put this down in writing.

Rules into Values

Personal, self-limiting rule	Unhelpful outcome of applying rule	Personal value behind rule	Flexible way of applying rule
I must never fail at anything	Puts a lot of pressure on me	I want to be a success at what I do	I should try to succeed at some things, but not all
I must always do my best to be liked by everyone	I am always over-thinking others' reactions to me	I want to be liked by those around me	It is okay to be disliked, as long as I consider my actions as kind and friendly
I must always put 100% into everything I do	When I am ill or busy, I can't keep to this rule and I feel awful	I want to be productive	I must recognise that there are many factors that impact performance
I must study others closely to make sure I am as good as them	It takes up a lot of my energy that could be better spent elsewhere	I want to be equal to others	It can be helpful to compare myself with others, but not at all times

Chapter 6. Experiments

Introduction

Many of the chapters in this book implicitly encourage the use of the scientific method. When you fill out a maintenance worksheet or record and reflect on your day in a diary, you are, in a sense, collecting data. When you challenge your thoughts, you do so by looking for evidence that will change your mind. This chapter continues this theme with models that propose hypotheses that can be tested using experiments. The more experiments you conduct that dispute your unhelpful beliefs, the more likely you are to be able to change them to better align with reality.

Behavioural Experiment (p.116) represents this idea perfectly. It suggests parameters for the experiment – what needs to happen for your prediction to come true, how much you believe in this prediction and so forth. Furthermore, it allows you to highlight what a more realistic prediction would look like and what helpful or unhelpful behaviours might swing the results either way. Finally, it encourages you to test out your expectations and record the outcome. Any result that you arrive at can then either reinforce your current beliefs or challenge them in a way that provides you with a more accurate mental map of the world. Imagery-Based Exposure (p.124) and the Resilience-Developing Model (p.118) both use this methodology in different ways to ensure that your beliefs can withstand being tested.

One of the most frequently used experiments in therapeutic treatments is graded exposure, which involves exposing yourself to evidence that your fears are unjustified. This is done in a gradual manner – you are encouraged to start small and then face progressively more difficult fears. This approach has been used with much success with phobias (see Graded Exposure for Phobias, p.130) but, like many other CBT-based treatments, it can be customised for other specific disorders (such as OCD Graded Exposure, p.132).

While this chapter is structured around the idea of experiments, not all the models presented here necessarily follow such a clear-cut format. Some, like Worry Time (p.120) or Stimulus Discrimination (p.122), actively encourage you to worry or imagine worst-case scenarios, in the full knowledge that you will have an adverse reaction. When your anxiety rises and negative physical symptoms appear, both models then ask you to stay with the feelings and understand that, while the situation is unpleasant, you are in no danger and actually do have control over what happens next. This realisation lies behind many of the experiments found in this chapter. The anticipated fear or anxiety you experience is almost always worse than the actual encounter. If it is not, then that might be a sign that the problem is not entirely psychological to begin with.

Going out into the world and conducting these experiments is not easy. There is a reason that this chapter comes later in this book. You will have to apply what you have learnt from formulating your problems and the motivation that you have gained from creating specific goals. You might even need the help of the relaxation strategies found in Chapter 3. These resources will help, and they can also be supplemented with cue cards, such as the ones found at the end of this chapter. Coping Cards (p.134) and Cognitive Cue Cards (p.136) allow you to carry with you a physical reminder of what you have learned, whether it is a list of your coping strategies or a list of your helpful thinking styles, so you can refer to them in distressing situations if needed.

Consider using the models in this chapter if you understand the nature of your problems but are still struggling to properly incorporate that learning into your life. It is one thing to know something in a theoretical sense; it is quite another to know it through lived encounters. Humans learn best through repeated experience. Sometimes it is necessary to put down your books and test out what you have learned. Only then can you truly see if these alternative explanations for your problems stand up to scrutiny.

6.1 Behavioural Experiment

Bennett-Levy, J., Butler, G., Fennell, M.J.V., Hackmann, A., Mueller, M. & Westbrook, D. (Eds.) (2004). *The Oxford handbook of behavioural experiments.* Oxford University Press.

Purpose

There are many ways to challenge your beliefs. Behavioural Experiment allows you to use your own recent experiences as evidence for a change in perspective. In many ways, this makes a lot of sense, as distressing past experiences often colour the way we see our present. If experience is responsible for the way we feel now, it stands to reason that new experiences that contradict our past ones might be the most effective way of conquering our current fears and cognitive distortions. We learn not just from reading or studying but from doing. Only then, after reflecting on the outcome of our experiment, can we see how unrealistic our initial beliefs were.

Suitability

This model is useful for people who want to challenge their beliefs not simply through analysis and thought-challenging but also through lived experience. While it is possible to see the truth of something through reflection, many people learn best by testing out their hypotheses in the real world. When your experiments succeed or fail, you can then use that knowledge to change any inaccurate beliefs you might have. Anyone can reinforce their learning through using Behavioural Experiment, but it works particularly well with people who have phobias or severe anxiety about certain situations.

How to use

Start by choosing a prediction that you want to test out. Write down on the worksheet what your prediction is, the situation it would occur in, how much you believe that the prediction will come true and how you will know if it comes true or not. Let's say you predict that, if you pet a particular dog, it will bite you. You now have the beginning of an experiment mapped out. By setting up your experiment in this way, you can be sure that success or failure can be accurately measured. Once you have set up your working hypothesis, list your behaviours that might make your prediction come true. Draw on past experience to give detail to this section and to make it clear to yourself how, occasionally, your own actions fulfil your fears.

Next, decide on a more realistic prediction of what might happen in this scenario. Has the dog ever bitten anyone else before? Has it ever growled at you? Wouldn't the dog's owner have trained the dog not to bite? Ask yourself these and similar questions to create a more realistic expectation of what would happen and write it down on the worksheet. It is fine if you don't believe this outcome to be true. After all, the whole purpose of conducting your experiment is to see whether this more realistic prediction is likely to be more true than your original prediction. Before moving on to actually pet the dog, reflect and write down what helpful behaviours you could adopt that would reduce your anxiety and improve the outcome.

After you have performed your experiment, return to the worksheet. What actually happened? Was it as you predicted originally, or closer to the more realistic one? Think about how it felt to behave differently. Did any of the helpful behaviours work? What did you learn from doing the experiment? There is usually a high chance that the more realistic prediction will come true, but occasionally the feared one will come true instead. The only way to discover if this is a statistical anomaly is to test out your original prediction again. If the realistic prediction still fails to happen, it might need reworking, or you might want to consider that the problem does not lie with you but with the unpleasant situation itself. Use the bottom half of the worksheet to describe what you have experienced and what it means to you.

Situation	My prediction	How much do I believe prediction will come true? %	How will I know if that prediction comes true?
I will speak up and voice my opinions in the next staff meeting	My ideas will be ignored or dismissed out of hand	80%	The conversation will rapidly move on

Behavioural Experiment

My unhelpful behaviours

I will speak too quietly and not make eye contact

I will agree with whatever someone says and not assert myself by disagreeing

A more realistic prediction would be...

My thoughts will get the same attention as others, although that does not mean that everyone will agree with what I have to say

My helpful behaviours

I will speak clearly and sit straight and tall

I will bring notes to the meeting so I will be able to quote facts to back up my points

What actually happened?	I brought up three points at the meeting and each was listened to and responded to in some detail
How much did my original prediction come true? %	30%
Which prediction was supported?	The realistic prediction was more accurate.
How did it feel to behave differently?	I felt going in with a plan made me confident. I also knew that I'd be writing it all down on this paper, so that motivated me
What did I learn from the experiment?	My behaviour plays an important part in how others receive my ideas. If I feel more confident, I am more likely to be listened to

6.2 Resilience-Developing Model

Padesky, C., & Mooney, K. (2012). Strengths-based cognitive-behavioural therapy: A four-step model to build resilience. *Clinical Psychology & Psychotherapy, 19*(4), 283–290.

Purpose

When we think of the term 'resilience', a few images may come to mind: toughness, armoured, ability to bounce back and weather storms. The Resilience-Developing Model understands resilience as the ability to adapt to life stresses. These might be traumatic life events, such as loss of loved ones, break-up of a long-term relationship, loss of job or home, or economic misfortune. Generally, we have little control over these events and have to accept and live through them. Being resilient means you are able to face these challenges, tolerate them and learn from them, without them fundamentally damaging your sense of self and worth.

Resilience is not something that you are born with, although genetic inheritance may give some people added ability to adapt. It is something that you develop over time, is very much rooted in early childhood and the instilling of inner confidence and sense of self from a secure upbringing, and is also something you can develop through experience of such losses and failures. In this way you learn that what doesn't kill you can make you stronger. This learning process can be fast-forwarded if you are willing to experiment with strategies that might help you develop resilience quicker. The Resilience-Developing Model is a helpful introduction to such strategies.

Suitability

If you find yourself in a distressing situation where there is little you can do to improve it right now, you will find it helpful to develop resilience strategies. These specific strategies can help you manage your own strong emotions, deal with difficult people, control unhelpful behaviour that might make the situation worse and avoid unproductive self-blame. The Resilience-Developing Model can be helpful for anyone who feels they are too easily overwhelmed by challenges and that they need to be better prepared and able to withstand them.

How to use

Look at your life and ask yourself where you could benefit from being more resilient. Is it in the workplace, within your family dynamic or in your romantic relationships? Write this down on the worksheet and then decide what strategies might help you build that resilience. These might include models and techniques described in this book, or they might involve behaviours or thinking patterns you have seen others use effectively in similar situations. Use your knowledge to list a few ideas. If any prove to be counterproductive, you can always replace them in the future.

Now ask yourself how you can apply these strategies to your own situation. Look to the future for any upcoming conflicts on the horizon. You might find that you will need to adapt some of your strategies, not simply to the context but also to your level of confidence in your own abilities. This is fine. It's important to take these steps gradually. Under 'How to apply strategies for this specific challenge', note down the ideas that come to mind.

Picture in your head what resilience would look like. Imagine how it would feel if you were to apply your strategies successfully. Visual imagery can be a powerful motivator. If you can envisage success, it can feel more attainable. Then set out to accomplish these strategies in the coming week. You might not be able to do all of them, but hopefully there will be enough opportunities to see the effect of some of them. Afterwards, return to the model and write down the results. What was the outcome of applying these resilience strategies? Notice if you were able to better manage your thoughts and behaviours and whether this had an influence on how you felt and acted.

Resilience-Developing Model

Where would you like to enhance your resilience?

I would like to be able to handle criticism better

Strategies to put into action	How to apply strategies for this specific challenge
Focus on my breathing when I get upset	Ask my mother-in-law how she would prefer that things are done and try to reach a compromise
Don't focus on the negative comments but instead on any constructive elements the criticism might include	Tell my relatives when they say hurtful things and don't accept their excuse that it is a 'cultural thing'
Understand that criticism of my actions is not criticism of me	Disengage from harmful criticism by changing the subject from me to a positive experience that I have shared with another
Accept that people sometimes accidentally say hurtful things	
Become better at challenging criticism if I feel it is unjust	Practise mindfulness exercises when I am criticised for being late; shrug it off
Know that the intensity of my emotions will decrease in time	

What would resilience look like?	It would look like me confronting a problem, not running away from it. It would be meeting others as an equal
How would resilience feel?	It would feel anxiety inducing at first, I'd be worried that I'd offend others. After a while I think I would feel empowered and more confident in my abilities

Results of applying strategies

I attempted to respond better to criticism from my family and in-laws this week. It had some success, but they accused me of being emotional. As I continue this, I will focus more on staying calm and breathing and not allowing my emotions to take over. When I did get criticism, it helped to be able to step back and give it a little perspective. It made me think that others might be critical of me, but that doesn't mean I have to see things their way

6.3 Worry Time

Borkovec, T.D., Wilkinson, L., Folensbee, R. & Lerman, C. (1983). Stimulus control applications to the treatment of worry. *Behaviour Research and Therapy, 21*(3), 247–251.

Purpose

When you are constantly worrying about the smallest things, you will eventually start to experience negative physical symptoms and emotions connected to anxiety. These symptoms might become a source of additional worry, and they will most certainly reduce your ability to cope with daily challenges. In these situations, it is important first to identify whether your worries are about things you can change or if they are outside your control. If you are unsure of this, you can use the Worry Diary (Chapter 4, p.70) to give you a little clarity.

Worries that are outside your control, sometimes called hypothetical worries, cannot be solved by problem-solving or planning a course of action. So you need a way to reduce the significance and importance that you attribute to them. This can be done by challenging any negative or positive stereotypes that you have about worry, such as the belief that, if you don't worry, terrible things will happen. Alternatively, you can use a model like Worry Time to control those aspects of your hypothetical worries that you do have power over: namely, when you worry and for how long. If the end result is to make your worries feel less overwhelming, being able to dictate when they occur can do much to reassert your confidence in managing them successfully.

Suitability

The Worry Time model is very helpful for people who have generalised anxiety disorder, are chronic worriers or are frequently preoccupied with hypothetical worries that are outside their control. Worry Time allows you to get some semblance of control back into your own hands. You might not be able to make your worries disappear, but you can restrict thinking about them to a set time, so they take up less headspace. Once you realise you can do this, you may find your confidence will increase. Your worries might not seem so overwhelming when you can consciously decide when and for how long you worry about them.

How to use

The Worry Time worksheet should be used daily. Ideally, you should aim to sit down and list your worries at the same time each day. Try to avoid doing this late at night as it is easy to then take your worries to bed with you. If you make Worry Time into a habit, it will be harder to find excuses to avoid it. It is essential that you do your best not to miss any days. I recommend that you spend 20–30 minutes on Worry Time initially, but as the weeks pass, if this begins to feel unnecessarily long, then make it shorter.

In your allocated time, write down any hypothetical worries that have crossed your mind in the past 24 hours. Once they are all on the worksheet, allow yourself to freely worry about them and entertain any catastrophic thoughts. It's a good idea to use a timer, so you know when your worry time is up. When the alarm goes off, put away the model, out of sight. Don't then go straight back to your day; instead, do something that you enjoy that will absorb your attention and signal to your brain that the time for worrying is now over.

Your hypothetical worries will return eventually, but instead of allowing your mind to dwell and ruminate on them, tell yourself that you will do so only at the next Worry Time. You are likely to find that, when you actually get to the next Worry Time, the importance of those worries might have faded, or you have forgotten about them completely. This is an important realisation to make. At the end of the week, reflect on this and note it down, with anything else relevant you have noticed, using the weekly worry review space provided.

Worry Time

My daily worry time is ___19:00___   **Length of time worrying** __20 mins__

- I worry that there will be an unforeseeable expense that I haven't budgeted for
- I'm worried that my son isn't working hard enough at school and this might eventually mean he doesn't get into a good university
- I worry that if I get sick that I won't be able to look after my family
- I worry that it's dangerous to go outside at night in my neighbourhood
- I worry that I will be late for appointments
- I am worried that others judge me for being a poor parent
- I am anxious that my children are studying my behaviour and becoming worriers themselves
- I worry that that my panic attacks will return

Post-worry time pleasurable activity

I will play with the children

Weekly worry review

I found that, when I sat down and wrote down the worries, they were not as intense as when I experienced them during the day. I found it hard to prevent myself from problem-solving those worries that were out of my control

6.4 Stimulus Discrimination

Foa, E.B. & Rothbaum, B.O. (1998). *Treating the trauma of rape: Cognitive-behavioral therapy for PTSD.* Guilford Press.

Purpose

One of the most distressing symptoms of PTSD is flashbacks. These are triggered by situations and sensory cues – sometimes quite minor details – that recall your traumatic experience and can make you feel that you are reliving it as the event unfolds with sickening realism in your mind. Your brain focuses on these harmless sensory cues, inflates them with significance, and derives from them intense anxiety and fear that you are currently in danger and need to act – either to fight or flee.

The Stimulus Discrimination model is designed to help you stay with and come through the flashbacks. It can help you bring yourself back to the present, away from those traumatic memories and worries about your safety. By standing your ground and labelling the differences between what is happening in the here and now and what belongs in your traumatic memories, you can collect enough evidence to convince yourself that you are not in harm's way. This strategy can teach your brain that perceived threats need to meet a certain evidential standard (your senses, body and mind all have to agree) before they deserve an extreme coping strategy such as fight or flight.

Suitability

This is a useful model for people who are vulnerable to symptoms of PTSD. When a flashback occurs, your senses trick you into believing you are reliving a traumatic experience. This distressing situation can be reversed by identifying the differences between the here and now and your memories. Stimulus Discrimination can train you to be able to do this. Many of us have experienced traumatic life events, but not all will lead to PTSD – some can be precipitating factors in other conditions, such as depression. This model is only recommended for people with specific PTSD symptoms, as it's unlikely to benefit you otherwise. If you are unsure what you are experiencing, I recommend that you consult a trained PTSD therapist.

How to use

First identify a recent flashback. Where were you? Who were you with? What was happening? Write these situational details down on the worksheet. Next, explore what that setting shared with your traumatic memory. You are looking for a particular sight, sound, smell and so on that might be responsible for triggering the flashback. It should not be difficult to identify as it's most likely that this sensory detail is very pronounced and lingers in your mind for some time.

After you have written down the similarities between the two situations, identify the differences. You should find that, despite one or two similar details, your situation is very different from the traumatic event itself. Use the prompts in the worksheet to highlight these differences. Once you have done this, write a reassuring statement analysing the situation, drawing on what you know about anxiety and its effects on the body and mind. The psychoeducation material in Chapter 3 can be a good refresher here. Memorise your statement for future use.

You can complete one of these worksheets each time you have a flashback, but the aim of this model is to equip you with the tools to reduce your anxiety when a flashback occurs. When the next one happens, try to recognise what your senses are telling you, and whether they contradict your initial assumptions about being in danger. Recite your reassuring statement and tell yourself that, just because you think you are in a place of danger does not mean that you really are. Consider using this worksheet alongside Grounding (Chapter 3, p.66) to help you redirect your attention from the past back to the present.

Experiments 123

Stimulus Discrimination

Situation/trigger

Walking down a stairwell to get to my car in the garage

Similarities

Then...
- Someone was in the stairwell
- Dark, poor lighting

Now...
- Someone was in the stairwell
- Dark, poor lighting

Differences

	Then...		Now...
Sight	It was a man waiting to attack someone		It was an old woman trying to climb up the stairs
Sound	Sniffing, sound of his bracelets		Sound of her walking stick
Smell	Sweat		Disinfectant smell
Taste	Blood in my mouth		N/A
Body	Fear, heart rate going fast, adrenaline rush		Nervous, compassion for old woman struggling
Knowledge	That I might die		That I am very unlikely to be attacked in the same place twice

Reassurance

I know that there is a difference between a perceived threat and an actual threat. I am able to list those things and identify the difference. My emotions are strong, but they are made stronger by the way that I interpret them. I am ultimately in control of how I think/act

6.5 Imagery-Based Exposure

Josefowitz, N. (2017). Incorporating imagery into thought records: Increasing engagement in balanced thoughts. *Cognitive and Behavioral Practice, 24*(1), 90–100.

Purpose

Traumatic memories can resurface in the form of flashbacks, nightmares and dissociative episodes. These can cause a great deal of anxiety and lead to behaviour that is out of character and that further reinforces the anxiety. While it might be easier in the short term to avoid these memories, it will do nothing to stop them recurring. If they are not dealt with effectively, your mental health can deteriorate and further situations might trigger your past trauma.

Imagery-Based Exposure is a technique that encourages you to face your anxiety instead of redirecting your attention elsewhere. It can be used to demonstrate that, while your thoughts can increase your anxiety and fear, they cannot harm you, and, unlike actual threats, they can be managed by focusing on them and recognising them for what they are – just thoughts. Ultimately, your present is different from your past and there will be plenty around you that justifies this conclusion. By avoiding your anxiety, you might only make it worse.

Suitability

Exposure to distressful situations can sometimes be so difficult that imagery work needs to be done before direct encounters can be attempted. This is even more relevant when the situation involves past trauma that cannot be directly revisited but still needs to be detached from present anxiety. Imagery-Based Exposure can be seen as the antithesis of Visual Imagery (Chapter 3, p.58), which applies visual imagery to reduce anxiety. This model uses imagery to increase anxiety so you learn that the negative physical symptoms that arise are due to your thinking process and not to any external forces. When you see that you have control over these symptoms, their hold over you will weaken.

How to use

Pick an upsetting or traumatic memory that has been regularly surfacing in the last few weeks. Expect your anxiety to increase when you bring your mind back. When the distress is at its peak, rate it on a scale of 0–100. Now explore the thoughts that came through your mind. They can be about the traumatic event or the aftermath. They can be perceptions of the event or judgements about yourself or others. Allow them free rein, but make sure to write them down as accurately as possible. Connect these thoughts with the emotions you feel right now. These might be reflections of what you felt during the traumatic event, but they also might be more complex and incorporate aspects from other areas.

While the memory is still present, write down what you felt like doing in response to this imagery exercise. Was it to focus on something else? Was it to run out of the room? Expect these reactions to surface, but do your best to focus on the task in hand. Write these responses down and then ask yourself what would have been the result if you had followed that urge. Would your anxiety have decreased? Almost certainly, but consider what that would have taught you about your anxiety – that the only way to deal with it is to redirect your attention elsewhere, even if that involves fleeing a harmless situation.

So, instead, sit with these thoughts and emotions and face them. Recognise where you are and the differences between then and now. Bring to your attention what you now know about the psychoeducation of anxiety and remind yourself that the strong feelings and physical symptoms that you are feeling can be managed. Keep doing this until you feel your level of distress decreases. Rate it again on a 0–100 scale and resolve to practise this exercise regularly.

Imagery-Based Exposure

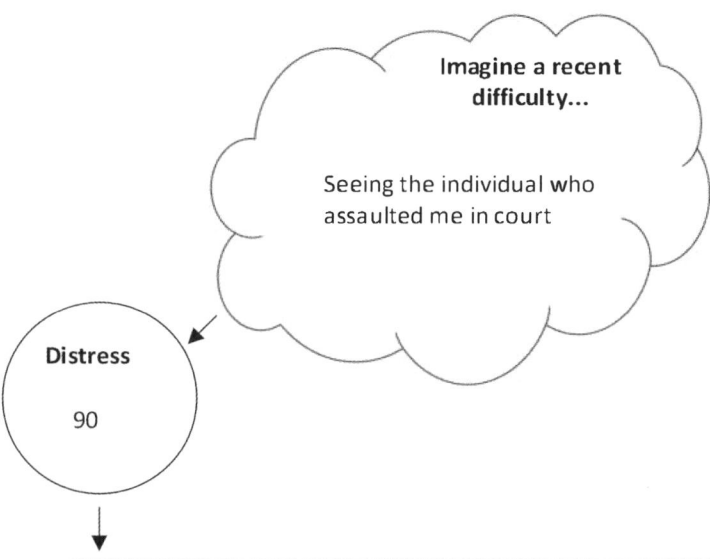

Imagine a recent difficulty...

Seeing the individual who assaulted me in court

Distress 90

What thoughts showed up in response to this memory?
It brought back the memory of the assault. I thought about how long the process had taken to get to this point, to have my day in court. I thought about what a senseless act it had been; that I didn't deserve what happened and I thought, 'Am I safe here? Could he still do something to me?'

What feelings and emotions showed up in response to this memory?
I felt helpless. I felt like everything I had done to testify could be undone and would be pointless. I felt angry that I had to go through this process and I felt tired and my head hurt

What did you feel like doing in response to this memory?
I felt like running away, getting as far away from the court as I could

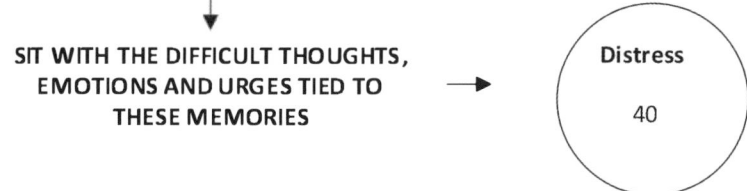

SIT WITH THE DIFFICULT THOUGHTS, EMOTIONS AND URGES TIED TO THESE MEMORIES → **Distress** 40

6.6 Downward Arrow Model

Beck, J.S. (2005). *Cognitive therapy for challenging problems: What to do when the basics don't work.* Guilford Press.

Purpose

Unhealthy core beliefs need to be named and understood before they can be tackled. For many people, these core beliefs remain obscure, their influence only discernible in automatic thoughts or maladaptive behaviour. However, by referring to these thoughts and the emotional/physiological reactions that follow, you can trace a route back to the fundamental beliefs that are having such an impact on how you see yourself, others and the world.

The Downward Arrow Model can help you quickly figure out what your core beliefs are. This process can be distressing, so it is important that you realise that, just because you hold a certain core belief, it does not in any way mean that the belief is objectively true. Many of the models in Chapter 5 can help you see how unhealthy core beliefs are maintained and how they can be successfully challenged.

Suitability

The Downward Arrow Model is an effective method for uncovering your core beliefs. It can be quite an emotionally taxing exercise, though, so I suggest you do it in a comfortable environment where you feel safe. Often, when you face the full significance of what your automatic thoughts hint at, you feel worse than when you started. Expect this and plan accordingly. Practise a few relaxation exercises after completing this model or do something that you enjoy. Many mental health issues are rooted in deeply held core beliefs and the short-term discomfort felt when doing this model can be outweighed by the benefit of knowing the source of your troubles.

How to use

Start by turning your attention to a recurring thought that provokes a strong emotional reaction. Note on the worksheet your reaction to this thought. How does your body respond? Ask yourself, if this thought were true, what would it say about you as a person? It might be a very self-critical thought. Try not to make excuses for it or push it to one side; instead, listen to your body and how it responds to this criticism. Often this self-critical thought will spiral further downwards: for instance, if you think that you are a poor driver, you might then think you are incompetent at most things, which in turn allows the further thought that you have no value as a person at all. Try not to phrase anything as a question; aim to define your beliefs in short, declarative sentences, such as, 'I am incompetent' or 'I have no value as a person'.

Much of this introspection work flies in the face of other material in this book. The aim here is not to understand how unhelpful thinking styles might make you feel worse, but to actively encourage your worst thoughts and doubts to come out so you can better understand them and where they come from. Once you can identify your unhelpful core beliefs, you can continue to do the hard work of challenging them and demonstrating that they are not an accurate reflection of who you are as a person.

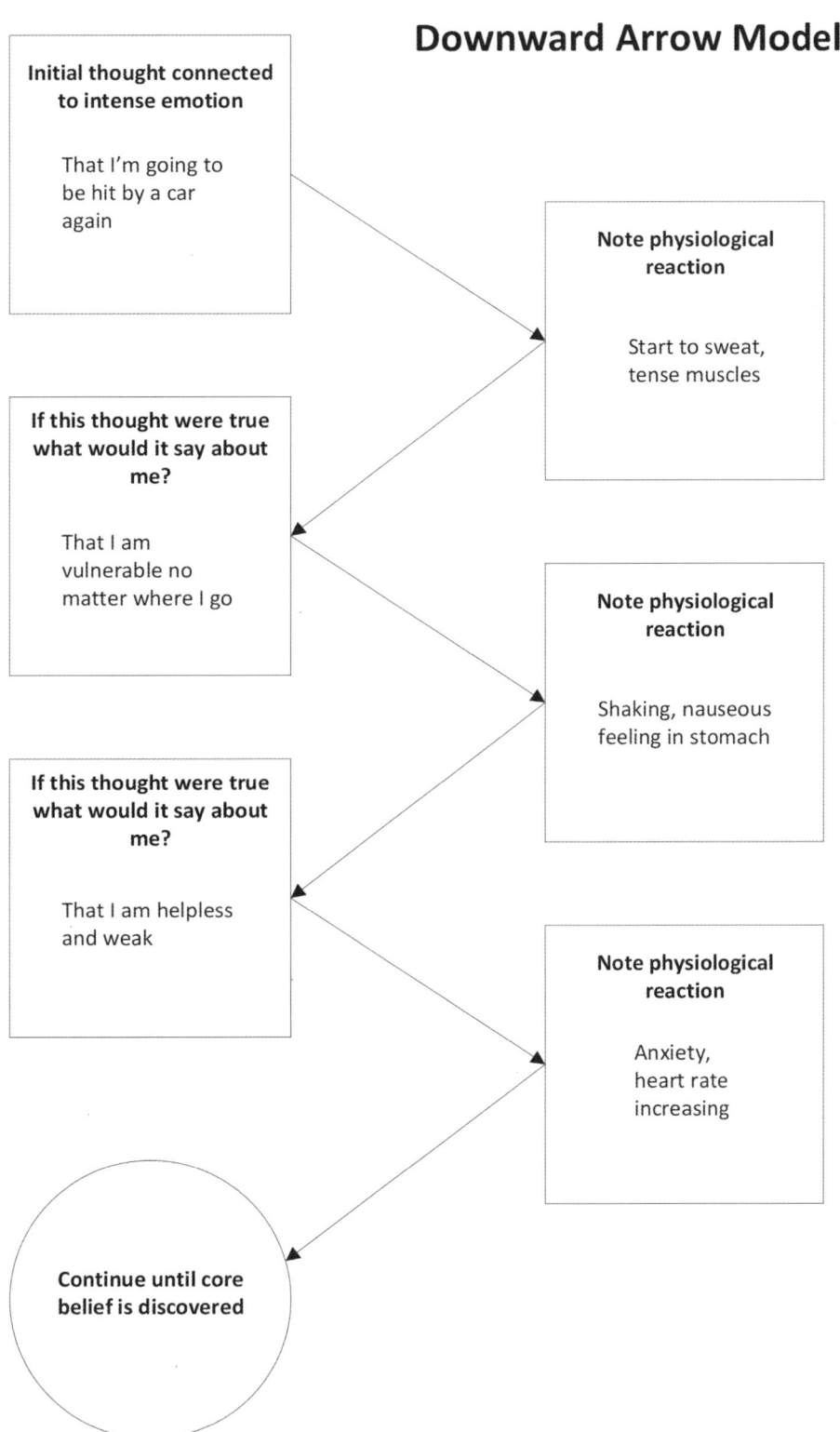

6.7 Core Belief Experiment

Bennett-Levy, J., Butler, G., Fennell, M.J.V., Hackmann, A., Mueller, M. & Westbrook, D. (Eds.) (2004). *The Oxford handbook of behavioural experiments*. Oxford University Press.

Purpose

Unhealthy core beliefs often lie at the heart of our suffering. While they can be successfully challenged by questioning our thinking process, nothing teaches better than experience. The Core Belief Experiment builds on that, in that it shows how our predictions about ourselves and others are often incorrect. This is chiefly because they rest on false premises: for example, they derive from core beliefs that have very little foundation in reality. These premises can be tested by creating experiments that challenge our assumptions. By repeatedly demonstrating to ourselves what poor judges of outcome we are, we can plant a seed of doubt that maybe some of those assumptions we have been carrying around for years are not as true as we have always thought.

Suitability

If you have discovered unhealthy core beliefs that are proving resistant to typical core belief-challenging techniques such as Core Belief Challenging (Chapter 5, p.106), you may find the Core Belief Experiment can offer an alternative. By encouraging you to design an experiment that tests whether your beliefs are valid, it enables you to collect evidence that demonstrates the invalidity of your former thinking and points you in the direction of more balanced core beliefs.

How to use

First, identify an unhealthy core belief that you want to challenge. If you are struggling with this, consider using the Downward Arrow Model (p.126) to help you identify the entrenched beliefs that may be causing your current difficulties. Create a task or experiment that allows you to test whether that core belief is true and write it down under 'Task' on the Core Belief Experiment worksheet. You might find that your core beliefs are very vague and difficult to translate into behaviours. It can sometimes help to consider the behaviours your core beliefs have discouraged you from doing. If you strongly believe you are inherently vulnerable, for example, doing something that has a slight element of danger might be a good way to initially challenge this central belief.

When you have your experiment in mind, write down your prediction on the worksheet. What do you expect will happen when you perform the task? Listen to any accompanying fear or anxiety but don't allow it to dissuade you from your goal. Complete the task, return to the worksheet and write down the results. Did what you predict come true? If there is a discrepancy between your prediction and reality, consider whether there have been similar incidents in the past where your dire predictions didn't come to pass. What does that say about the accuracy of the underlying beliefs that influenced those predictions? Write down any reflections in the space for 'Conclusions'. Use this worksheet and any other core belief exercises you have been practising to revise your unhealthy core belief into something more balanced that better reflects your actual experience.

It isn't easy to challenge core beliefs. If you are tempted to dismiss the accumulating evidence against them, repeat the exact experiment. Does the outcome change significantly? Probably not. Remind yourself that you are very likely to meet resistance when trying to create a more balanced core belief, but that resistance is evidence in itself that you are heading in a direction that might alleviate your suffering.

Core Belief Experiment

Core belief
I am useless

Task
To help out at a local fundraiser, e.g. handing out badges, selling drinks, etc.

Prediction
That I will not be able to do the tasks asked of me without getting flustered and breaking down

Result
I was able to do all of the tasks. Though I was anxious for a lot of the time, I did not need to take any breaks and I was thanked for contributing afterwards

Conclusion
I had everything explained to me in advance, so I was able to pick up on what I needed to do relatively fast. I felt useful, but at the same time what I was doing was very simple

Balanced core belief
I can do some things well. I am not entirely useless. Perhaps I need to find challenges that are at an appropriate level for my abilities, not too easy, not too hard

6.8 Graded Exposure for Phobias

McLean, P.D. & Woody, S.R. (2001). *Anxiety disorders in adults: An evidence-based approach to psychological treatment.* Oxford University Press.

Purpose

Phobias can range from fears of dogs and heights to fears of people and enclosed spaces. The list of individual phobias is truly staggering and can account for a wide number of irrational, persistent and excessive fears. Fortunately, all phobias can be dealt with in a similar way, with graded exposure. Graded exposure simply involves slowly reintroducing the feared activity back into your life in small, incremental steps. It may be almost impossible to convince someone who is afraid of enclosed spaces to step into a lift. But if they decide to work on their fear by progressively exposing themselves to smaller and smaller rooms, they will find that eventually they can use a lift and cope with their fears.

Suitability

Graded exposure is an effective method for reducing irrational fears. The more you expose yourself to fears, the quicker those fears will become less intense and the more confident you will become in your coping abilities. Consider using this model after you have completed the Phobia Ladder (Chapter 2, p.42) and want to challenge phobias such as claustrophobia, agoraphobia and other excessive fears that can easily become overwhelming.

How to use

Start Graded Exposure for Phobias by choosing some activities, objects, creatures or environments that you are afraid of. Don't choose anything that presents too much difficulty, but don't choose anything that doesn't provoke much fear either. List them on the worksheet. Use the 0–100 scale provided to roughly measure how much anxiety you might have. If the activity scores less than 30, consider finding something a little more challenging. If it is higher than 80, you should probably to work your way up to that level by selecting some easier challenges first.

Once you have a list of feared activities, set out to accomplish them one by one. Use the worksheet to record the date, time and your starting level of anxiety. Expose yourself to the feared activity and be sure to keep your attention fixed on it. Your mind is likely to start catastrophising and you will notice the fight/flight response kicking in. Sit with these emotions and don't run away from them. Tell yourself that, no matter how you feel, you are in no danger, and that, while high levels of anxiety can be distressing, they won't harm you. If it helps, focus on your breathing and try to slow it down (see Square Breathing Technique (Chapter 3, p.56). Use this to manage your anxiety – but don't use it as an avoidance strategy.

As you expose yourself to the feared activity and nothing bad happens, you should start to see your anxiety slowly decrease. When it is reaches 0 or close to that number, you can stop the exercise. It is important not to stop the exercise before this moment as that would reinforce the validity of your fear and make the next attempt even more difficult.

Record on the worksheet how long it took and any reflections that come to mind – what you found helpful or unhelpful, for example. You can use these reflections to compare the exercise with past instances where you faced your fears and acted differently. Finally, congratulate yourself on what you have accomplished and plan another exposure exercise for the next day. Try to ensure that it is a little more challenging than the last but still well within your capabilities.

Graded Exposure for Phobias

Date/time	Feared activity	Starting anxiety	Anxiety at end	Reflections	Duration
14/01/2022 – 14:00	Taking the bus into town with my partner	60	30	I had done this previously last week, so knew what to expect. My anxiety was reasonably high	20mins
15/01/2022 – 11:00	Taking the bus into town with my partner	50	20	My previous experience helped me realize that I do have control of my attention	15mins
16/01/2022 – 15:00	Taking the bus alone	70	20	It was tough to ride the bus alone as I couldn't talk to my partner. It took longer to relax	25mins
18/01/2022 – 21:00	Using the metro at night	80	30	I was so scared I almost did not attempt the exercise. Nothing terrible happened though	40mins

Target end anxiety

0 — 50

Anxiety too high for attempt

100

6.9 OCD Graded Exposure

Hezel, D.M., & Simpson, H.B. (2019). Exposure and response prevention for obsessive-compulsive disorder: A review and new directions. *Indian Journal of Psychiatry*, *61*(1), 85–92.

Purpose

While most mental health problems will result in your behaviour changing, with OCD those changes are not only more noticeable but also more debilitating. Compulsive behaviour can occupy hours of your time and drastically reduce the quality of your life. To reduce the urgency and need to perform your compulsions, you should start by questioning what impact they have. Do compulsions stop terrible things from happening, or do they simply reduce your anxiety? OCD Graded Exposure is designed to help you persuade yourself that the latter is the more believable by drawing attention to what happens when you don't act compulsively. Its experimental structure allows you to come to your own conclusions about what your actions are and are not responsible for.

Suitability

This is a very good model to help people with OCD prove to themselves that their compulsions do not keep them safe and only reduce their anxiety. OCD Graded Exposure can be used to face your obsessions and find better ways of relieving your acute anxieties, not through compulsive behaviour but either through redirecting attention or thought challenging (see Worry Tree (Chapter 5, p.100) and Thought-Disputing Model (Chapter 5, p.94)). This model is suitable for people who are at the point where they understand that obsessions and compulsions are symptoms of extreme anxiety and not practical solutions to ensuring their safety. As such, it should be used only after such tools as the Cognitive Model of Obsessive-Compulsive Disorder (Chapter 1, p.12) and Intrusive Thoughts Diary (Chapter 4, p.84) have been properly explored.

How to use

The OCD Graded Exposure worksheet can be divided into two halves: planning, and then reflection on the outcome of your plans. Begin by choosing an upcoming situation or event that you are fairly sure will trigger obsessive thoughts and compulsive behaviour. The more control you have over the situation, the better. If it involves other people, make sure that they are aware of what you are attempting and that they have agreed to be involved. Score this situation on the worksheet on a scale from 0–100, where the higher the number, the more anxiety you expect to feel. Write down your predictions of what will happen. These might be the specific thoughts that enter your head and the behaviours that you engage in when the anxiety begins to rise.

Now place yourself in the chosen situation and refrain from enacting any of your compulsive behaviours. If, for instance, your compulsion is to check you have locked your front door when leaving your house, leave the house, close the door behind you, move a short distance away and don't go back to check that it is locked. Rate your anxiety at the start of this exercise. It might be quite high to begin with, but the longer you stand there, the more your anxiety levels should fall. Remind yourself that you did the lock the door and that any catastrophic thoughts you are having are not based on a realistic assessment of the situation. Under no circumstances should you check the lock on the door to reduce your anxiety, as to do so will undermine the point of the experiment.

When your anxiety has reduced significantly – below 20–30 – go back to the worksheet and record the outcome. What conclusions can you reach? Did your feared outcome occur? If you and your loved ones are still safe and your house unburgled, explore what that means about your predictions and beliefs. Score from 0–100 the strength of your belief that your compulsions are necessary. Record this on the worksheet. Hopefully, every time you perform these experiments, you should see that score decrease and feel more confident in your ability to distinguish between actual and perceived dangers.

OCD Graded Exposure

Situation	Expected anxiety %	What do you predict will happen?	Starting anxiety %	Anxiety at end %	Outcome: what actually happened?	Belief strength %
Leaving the house without checking the electrical outputs	70%	That my house will catch fire	80%	40%	I left the house without checking. I was anxious while away, but nothing disastrous happened	60%
Skipping my evening prayers	60%	That something misfortunate will happen to my family	40%	30%	My daughter tripped and fell, grazing her knee, but she wasn't seriously hurt	80%
Cooking a meal without washing my hands thoroughly	60%	I will give myself and others food poisoning	90%	30%	The meal was excellent and in the coming days no one was ill	30%

6.10 Coping Cards

Wright, J. (2006). Cognitive behavior therapy: Basic principles and recent advances. *FOCUS: The Journal of Lifelong Learning in Psychiatry, 4*(2), 173.

Purpose

This book contains an assortment of therapeutic models, worksheets and diaries that can be used in a variety of situations to deal with distress. It can be difficult to know or remember which to use in which situations, especially as certain situations will call for specific methods. Coping Cards are a handy way of reminding you of your coping strategies, both those that you are currently using successfully and those that you imagine will provide more support but you have yet to experiment with. You can carry these cards with you and refer to them when necessary. Also, having something physical like a card to hold can act as a reminder of all the progress that you have made to identify your difficulties and come up with productive solutions. It's easy to forget this when your fight/flight response is engaged and you are looking for any kind of escape.

Suitability

You can use Coping Cards to remind yourself of non-therapeutic coping strategies that you have used successfully in the past to feel better. Alternatively, you can use them as prompts for some of the therapeutic techniques you've learned from this book. They are a handy way of accessing solutions to your problems when you are feeling anxious or very low. They are suitable for anyone, but those who often feel overwhelmed by their emotions or who feel that their existing coping strategies might be hard to change should find them even more valuable.

How to use

Fill out a number of these cards so that when distressful situations occur you have something to fall back on to remind you how to better manage your problems. Choose situations that provoke strong emotional reactions and that you anticipate you will face in the near future. Then list the possible coping strategies you can use to improve your mood. These might include relaxation techniques (Chapter 3), thought disputing (Chapter 5) or redirecting your attention towards activities that give you a sense of mastery and control (Chapter 2). Not all the strategies need be strictly therapeutic – often a saying or a prayer that means a lot to you can have a powerful impact, and these can be written down on the cards as well.

When listing these strategies, be sure to ask yourself whether they are actual solutions to your problems or if they are maintaining the very problems you are trying to deal with. Someone who is experiencing social anxiety, for example, might cope by avoiding social situations where they might feel judged. It is unlikely that they would write this down on a card: it is no doubt something that they can remember to do without prompting, but, more importantly, it may be because their coping device may reinforce the fear that all social situations will involve judgement and so must be avoided at all costs. Have a good look at some of the techniques that you think might reduce your distress and only include those that have clear long-term benefits.

Coping Cards

The next time I am in <u>an anxiety-inducing</u> situation, I can

Remind myself of the flight/flight response

Focus attention on my breathing and away from the source of perceived danger

Take a sip of water and concentrate on how it tastes and feels

---

The next time I am in <u>a hopeless, ruminating</u> situation, I can...

Look at my diary and either follow what is in it or do something that will refocus my attention elsewhere

Do an activity that normally gives me pleasure or a sense of achievement

Call someone close to me and focus the conversation on their issues

---

The next time I am in _____ situation, I can...

The next time I am in _____ situation, I can...

6.11 Cognitive Cue Cards

Wright, J. (2006). Cognitive behavior therapy: Basic principles and recent advances. *FOCUS: The Journal of Lifelong Learning in Psychiatry, 4*(2), 173.

Purpose

We are often our own fiercest critics. We judge ourselves far more harshly than we do others, and by holding ourselves to a higher standard or magnifying our failures, we engage in a destructive cycle of self-criticism. Recognising this self-criticism might be easy when we are feeling in a calmer state, but in the midst of intense emotion it can be a struggle to balance our thoughts and be kind to ourselves. Cognitive Cue Cards can be used as a reminder of previous negative thoughts and how we were able to reinterpret them after the event. If your current situation has any parallels, you can draw on your previous insights to help you deal with your inner critic and resolve your present difficulties.

Suitability

Cognitive Cue Cards can be helpful for people with a very vocal inner critic that downplays their achievements and puts them down. They are a handy, readily accessible way of reminding yourself that there are other ways of interpreting a situation that do not necessarily involve self-criticism. They do this by presenting more balanced thoughts based on a combination of evidence of past successes and your innate coping abilities and self-worth. The cards can be used by anyone, but those experiencing depression might find them useful in combating negative thoughts brought on by episodes of low mood.

How to use

Consider the last few weeks and write down on the cue cards any distressful situations that caused negative thinking. You might want to return to some of your completed formulations in Chapter 1 if you are finding it difficult to recollect any. Notice how the cards use a situational trigger leading to a negative automatic thought – similar, for instance, to the Cognitive Maintenance Model (Chapter 1, p.6). This will help you ground your negative thought in a particular lived experience and reduce the idea that these thoughts come from nowhere and that you are powerless to stop them occurring.

Use the 'I know...' and 'It is true because...' prompts to reinterpret those situations now that time and emotional distance separate you from them. Come up with a competing vision that argues against your initial negative thought. For example, identify any unhelpful thinking styles that you've used or adopt a more compassionate view of yourself. Provide evidence for why this vision makes more sense than your initial negative thoughts. Once you have completed a number of these cards, carry them with you and, if a similar situation or thought arises, redirect your attention to them and reflect that, if you were able to create a more balanced thought last time, what prevents you from doing the same now?

Cognitive Cue Cards

Just because...
I was criticised at work
doesn't mean...
I am terrible at my job
I know...
that I am a competent and hard working employee
is true because...
of my proven track record of work accomplishments and successes

---

Just because...
I was unable to do everything that I set out to do today
doesn't mean...
I am lazy or useless
I know...
I can be productive
is true because...
I am juggling academic work, part-time employment and childcare all at the same time

---

Just because...

doesn't mean...

I know...

is true because...

Just because...

doesn't mean...

I know...

is true because...

Chapter 7. Interpersonal strategies

Introduction

Meaningful change comes from within us and from questioning our behaviour and thoughts. But it would be misleading to see ourselves as living in a bubble and not accept that our relationships with others have a significant impact on how we feel. While the other chapters in this book do not neglect the role of others, they tend to emphasise the self as the starting point on any journey of discovery. This chapter puts relationships with others centre stage and is intended for people who have found that a lot of their problems arise from unhealthy relationship dynamics and who are motivated to change them.

When trying to understand our relationships, a good place to begin is by looking at what we hope to get from our interactions with others. We all have a number of emotional and relationship needs, and being honest about whether those needs are being met can be the first step to recognising what needs to change. Acknowledging Needs (p.140) can help here, as can Circle of Contact (p.148), as it too invites you to take a closer look at your current situation. Using these models can make you aware of the support systems available to you and also highlight any deficiencies that might be present.

Often our difficulties with others can lead us to the realisation that our behaviour is either too passive or too aggressive – or, because we find it difficult to express ourselves, we swing from one to the other, sometimes with extreme consequences. If we are too passive, people may take advantage of us; if we are too aggressive, people may avoid us and we begin to feel isolated. Using the Thought Record for Assertiveness (p.142) can encourage reflection on our thoughts and behaviour preparatory to shifting them towards a more assertive style of communicating. This can then be reinforced by practising assertiveness techniques, as detailed in the Assertiveness Technique Log (p.144). While no one is assertive all the time, small changes here and there can make a difference to how we interact with others so as to avoid unintended consequences.

In our relationships with partners or close family members, we can often get stuck in patterns of behaviour that make us feel frustrated. They act in a certain way, and we respond in a way that triggers a predictable response from them. These patterns can become so ingrained that it can be difficult to see how they could be changed. The worksheets in this chapter are designed to help you identify these patterns and consider how you might reduce future conflict by changing a specific behaviour or way of interpreting a situation. In some cases, conflicts occur because emotions are high, and we do not give ourselves or others space or time to weigh our words carefully. Adding structure to conversations can be a way to give everyone the freedom to say what is on their mind without the fear of being aggressively challenged. A model such as Temperature Reading (p.146) can provide that structure until its benefits are absorbed and it starts to come more naturally to you.

As you explore the models in this chapter, it is important that you understand how much or how little you are responsible for a communication breakdown. If you are by nature very introspective, you may spend a lot of time looking for faults in yourself to explain why you are having such difficulties in your interpersonal relationships. There may, indeed, be work that you can do to improve how you behave, but in some cases, such as abusive relationships, there is instead a need to recognise the toxicity of the relationship and understand that you can't be held responsible for the problems of others. Consider using the Responsibility Pie (p.150) to challenge your automatic thoughts in these respects.

The models in this chapter are designed to help you explore how your behaviour and thoughts affect your relationships. In this sense, it is little different from the preceding chapters. A strong circle of friends and family can offer protection from stressful life events, so anything you can do to maintain and build on your relationships should bring rich rewards.

7.1 Acknowledging Needs

Maslow, A.H. (1943). A theory of human motivation. *Psychological Review, 50*(4), 370–396.

Purpose

The psychologist Abraham Maslow first proposed the idea that all humans have a common hierarchy of needs: basic needs, then psychological needs and, finally, self-fulfilment needs. Building on this, Acknowledging Needs is a model that can help you recognise what you need in order to lead a fulfilling life. The emphasis here is on relational needs, as this is often where people tend to put others' needs before their own, or disregard them.

Exploring your physical, emotional and relational needs can put you back in touch with what you want in the relationships in your life. This might bring about the realisation that your relationships are failing to meet those needs, and that change will be necessary to improve the quality of your life. Such changes are not likely to be easy, so it is crucial that you have a clear idea of what you want to achieve and why before setting out on that journey.

Suitability

This model is a great way of quickly exploring your needs and bringing your attention to those that you may have overlooked and neglected. In particular, exploring your emotional and relational needs can allow you to assess whether your current environment is meeting them all. Often this exploration can uncover discrepancies between your life now and the life you would like to be leading. People experiencing relationship difficulties will find this model particularly helpful to identify where they would like to see change, in themselves and in others.

How to use

Start the worksheet by listing your physical needs – shelter, food, safety and so forth. Be specific with what you see as a need. One person might simply see having a bed and roof over their head as enough; others might need more elaborate accommodation.

In the next section, list your emotional needs. An emotional need is something that is necessary for your emotional equilibrium. This list might include financial independence and security, a sense of community and a desire to do good in the world. You might find that some of your emotional needs are tied to your relational needs. This is to be expected as even the most introverted among us are still, deep down, social creatures.

Use the last section to explore what you need in your relationships with others. There might be a mix of emotional and physical needs here – honesty and hugs, for example. Do not be too concerned about disentangling them – just focus on your highly personal needs from others.

When you have finished this exercise, look at all the needs you have listed and identify where you feel your needs are met and where there may be deficits. You may wish to consider how those needs could be better met.

Acknowledging Needs

Physical needs

- Shelter
- Food
- Exercise
- Safety
- Sleep
- Money

Emotional needs

- A feeling of competence
- Self-compassion
- Sense of achievement in my work
- Purpose in life
- An idea of who I am and what I stand for
- Autonomy

Relationship needs

- Respect from others
- Warmth in relationships
- Love
- Others to confide in
- Romance
- Humour and a release from the stress of life

7.2 Thought Record for Assertiveness

Heimberg, R.G. & Becker, R.E. (1981). Cognitive and behavioral models of assertive behavior: Review, analysis and integration. *Clinical Psychology Review*, *1*(3), 353–373.

Purpose

Being assertive is about finding a balance between aggression and passivity. Someone who acts aggressively will put themselves first and ignore the wants and needs of others. A passive person will go along with the demands of others and, even if they believe differently, they will not voice their dissent. Passive behaviour can erupt into aggression over time, as all the pent-up anger escalates and some small, insignificant incident sets it off, with negative impacts on relationships with others.

The Thought Record for Assertiveness can be used to identify these passive and aggressive behaviours and thoughts and work out how to replace them with assertiveness. An assertive stance recognises that others are important and have needs that may be different from yours, but does not put them above your own needs. An assertive person stands up for themselves but doesn't seek to change or control the behaviour of others. This model will help you reflect on your own thoughts and behaviours and see where on this spectrum you currently stand.

Suitability

This is a useful model for anyone who believes that their behaviour is either too aggressive, too passive, or fluctuates between those two extremes. By helping you describe and analyse your behaviours and thoughts, this model can highlight where and how you may need to change your thinking and behaviour to improve your relationships with others.

How to use

First, describe on the worksheet a recent situation that involved you acting in an overly aggressive or passive manner. Describe the situation in detail, focusing on the time, the place, who you were with and what happened. Next, record what your emotional reaction was and any physical symptoms you noticed. Then describe your behaviour in response to the situation. You need to focus on your behaviour at the time, not later. For instance, if you were criticised at work, did you sit quietly and take the criticism, even though you believed it to be unfair, or did you start criticising your colleague in retaliation? Consider whether your behaviour was passive, assertive or aggressive, using the descriptions above.

Turn now to your thoughts and begin by listing those that you had at the time. Give each thought a belief rating from 0–100. The higher the number, the more you currently believe that a particular thought is true. Explore whether these thoughts are passive, assertive or aggressive. Passive thoughts will often put down your own performance or abilities; aggressive thoughts will criticise or attack the competency of others; an assertive thought strikes a balance between the two and sees your value while not disqualifying that of others. You will probably find you have recorded a mix of thoughts that vary in belief strength. Being able to see these thoughts written down can help you identify the thoughts that might be worth questioning and revaluating in order to behave more assertively in this relationship. Consider combining this with Thought-Disputing Model (Chapter 5, p.94) or Cost/Benefit Analysis (Chapter 5, p.98).

Interpersonal strategies   143

Thought Record for Assertiveness

Situation

My partner criticised my cooking

	Emotions	Physical symptoms	Behaviour
	Upset, frustrated, annoyed at her	Teary, dryness in throat	Apologised for the food

Thoughts	Belief	Type
I am a terrible cook	70	Passive
My partner is ungrateful and unkind	40	Aggressive
I shouldn't get so emotional over these comments	80	Passive
I am useless at everything	50	Passive
My partner and I need to rework our cooking arrangements	40	Assertive

Was this behaviour?

Passive   Assertive   Aggressive

7.3 Assertiveness Technique Log

Butler, G. & Hope, T. (2007). *Manage your mind: The mental fitness guide*. Oxford University Press.

Purpose

The purpose of the Assertiveness Technique Log is to record instances where you successfully use specific assertiveness techniques. These techniques can be briefly summarised as:

- **Basic assertion** – a clear statement that expresses your needs, wants and beliefs. It is a simple way to disclose what is important to you and is often framed as an 'I...' statement.
- **Empathetic assertion** – a compassionate statement that appreciates that others might not feel the same way that you do, but nevertheless you still need to express yourself.
- **Consequence assertion** – a strong statement that suggests that, if the other person is unwilling to listen to you, you will have to follow through with certain consequences. To be used sparingly.
- **Discrepancy assertion** – a method whereby you point out a discrepancy between what was previously said to you and what is being said now. An assertion that appeals to others' sense of rationality.
- **Negative feelings assertion** – a way of communicating how you are feeling and making the other person recognise how they are contributing to your emotional state.

All these techniques can be used to express yourself in a way that avoids excessive aggression or passivity. Doing so will help others realise that your voice is just as important as theirs. Hopefully this will reduce conflicts and your assertiveness will come not from a place of weakness but from a belief that you deserve to be heard as much any other person.

Suitability

The Assertiveness Technique Log is going to help you if you have recognised that a lack of assertiveness is at the core of many of your relationship difficulties. Once you have made that realisation, the next step is to begin practising assertiveness techniques and logging your attempts, using the model. By reflecting on your practice, you can see where you have developed your assertiveness skills and what still needs refining. Acting assertively does not always come naturally, but with practice it is possible to see significant improvement in a short space of time.

How to use

Once you have memorised the above assertion techniques, you need to go out and practise them on others. I suggest you start with the basic and empathetic assertion techniques, as they are the simplest to apply and will quickly produce results. Keep in mind that others may not always respond kindly to your assertiveness. If, for instance, you have always acted very passively, those close to you might misunderstand your assertiveness as an attack on them and become defensive. If this happens, the easiest way to resolve it is to be honest and tell them what you are doing. If you give them a rationale for your behaviour, they are less likely to take your comments personally and might even see the wisdom in what you are doing. It might be difficult at first to know whether you are being assertive or aggressive if others are reacting unpredictably. Try not to judge your assertive behaviour based on how other respond to it, but on whether your behaviour clearly expresses your needs while respecting the needs of others.

Each time you use these skills, record your attempts on the worksheet. Describe the techniques used, the situations and any reflections that occur to you. The more consciously you practise these techniques, the quicker they will become second nature.

Assertiveness Technique Log

Date/time	Technique used	Situation and how technique was used	Things to remember for next time
12/08/ 2022 14:00	Basic assertion	My friend wanted to stay longer at the shopping mall, but I made it clear that I had to go home	Did my best to emphasise 'I' statements but need in the future to use a firmer tone
15/08/ 2022 11:00	Empathic assertion	My mother wanted me to do run an errand for her but I explained that I had some studying to do	It worked well, but I ended up compromising and running the errand for her later
15/08/ 2022 19:00	Consequence assertion	My colleague said he was too busy to help me with a task we had both been given. I explained that it would get back to our boss if it was not done	I felt as if I was forcing him to help me, even though I knew he should be helping me on his accord

7.4 Temperature Reading

Satir, V., Banmen, J., Gerber, J. & Gomori, M. (1991). *The Satir model: Family therapy and beyond.* Science and Behavior Books.

Purpose

The Temperature Reading model is derived from the work of Virginia Satir, a family therapist who wanted to create a tool that would encourage more open and expressive communication between loved ones. By using a mix of conversational prompts, Temperature Reading can create a structured way of having difficult conversations so that one person does not feel overwhelmed by another and conflicts can be resolved through productive dialogue.

Suitability

Temperature Reading should be used by those who are having frequent relational difficulties with partners, close friends or family members. The structure it offers can make difficult conversations easier. It also creates a space where you can show others how you feel and how you appreciate their efforts. If you decide to use the model on a daily basis, it can work in a very similar way to Worry Time (Chapter 6, p.120), in that, by discussing any disagreements at a set time, rather than in the heat of the moment, you give yourself space to evaluate your thoughts, so that when you come to fill out the worksheet, you are less upset and more open to their point of view.

How to use

Is there someone with whom you are often in conflict? They might be a family member or an intimate partner or close friend. Ask them if they are interested in resolving some of the difficulties you are both having. If they are willing, decide on a regular time each day or each week to practise Temperature Reading. Whether you do a reading every day or every week is up to you, but if you are having daily arguments and fights, it is worth doing it every day to begin with. Later, when progress has been made, you can reduce it to once a week.

At the agreed time, sit down together and work your way through the worksheet. Start with 'Appreciations': share something that you have recently appreciated them doing. Then ask them if there is anything you have done that they have appreciated. Try to stick with this back-and-forth dialogue, where one person shares something uninterrupted and then invites the other to have their say – return to it if you stray.

Next, tell them what you want to say ('New information'). This might be bad news or something you think might be upsetting for them to hear. Try to keep to one point and to listen to their response but avoid becoming trapped in an argument. Follow the same process for 'Puzzles'. Focus on one thing they have done recently that puzzled you. Calling it a puzzle can make the conversation less confrontational and more collaborative, as it invites them to figure out with you why such and such happened. Follow this up with 'Recommendations for change'. These are not demands or ultimatums – just a way of sharing the changes in their behaviour that you would appreciate. This can be the most difficult step to complete as few people like to have their behaviour criticised, but by now you should have done the groundwork to sustain an amicable exchange of viewpoints.

Finish by sharing with each other your wishes, hopes and dreams for the future. These do not have to be related to the changes you want to see in each other; it's better if you focus on wider goals that remind you of the value of the relationship to you both. Often when a relationship is under stress, these values become less apparent, which is why it is so important to remind yourself of them on a regular basis. Try to capture accurately the essence of what you each say in the model, as writing it down can give your words more weight and a permanence that extends beyond the exercise itself.

Temperature Reading

	Myself	Name_____
Appreciations	This week I really appreciated the effort that you made in doing the washing up without being prompted. I also appreciated you booking a table for a meal out on Friday	
New information	I wanted to let you know about the new work hours that I will be doing. They might cause some disruption to our plans	
Puzzles	I was puzzled when you told me that you were going to be going abroad for a conference on such short notice	
Recommendations for change	I would like it if you were able to share your schedule with me in advance so I can prepare better. I would like you to help me with the childcare more now my work hours have changed	
Wishes, hopes and dreams	I am looking forward to our early retirement plans and I am dreaming of our holiday this summer when we can get away from the stress of our jobs	

7.5 Circle of Contact

DiClemente, C.C., Schlundt. D. & Gemmell, L. (2004). Readiness and stages of change in addiction treatment. *American Journal of Addiction, 13*(2),103–119.

Purpose

We often take our social support system for granted. While it changes and transforms as we grow, it remains a constant presence, and we can easily overlook its importance. Circle of Contact is an exercise to help us recognise the roles others play in our lives. It can highlight what others bring to our life and wellbeing or point us towards areas of deficit. Often, when we are feeling low, we isolate ourselves and push others away and subsequently feel all the more alone. Identifying that we are not alone and that we can make changes in how we conduct our relationships is an ideal first step towards re-engaging with the world.

Suitability

This model can help you understand the range and depth of your social relationships. Circle of Contact is for you if you tend to have low self-esteem and underestimate the importance of the meaningful relationships you have built over the years. Likewise, if you tend to downplay your closeness to others, the model can highlight that unhelpful thinking style. And if any of the circles in the worksheet are empty, it can prompt you to make addressing that a priority.

How to use

Begin with the Circle of Intimacy at the centre, and write down the names of the people in your life who you feel close to and can talk to about life's most meaningful subjects. These are people you may have spent years developing your relationships with and who you believe can be relied on if you are ever in need. Move outwards to the Circle of Friendship. Here, list people who you are close to and can talk openly with but perhaps not to the same depth and intimacy. In the Circle of Participation, write the names of people you do things with but then go your separate ways. Work colleagues, special interest and hobby group members and distant relatives might go in this circle. Finally, use the Circle of Exchange to list the people you see in passing on a regular basis and where some familiarity has been established but you have no relationship outside these exchanges. They might be someone working in your local cafe, or a neighbour you meet each morning as you walk to the bus stop. You may not even know their name. No matter how little your emotional connection with them, record them here, as they provide an important sense of community and belonging.

Once you have completed all the circles, reflect on what it looks like. Is this what you expected to see when you started the exercise? Are you surprised by anything? Keep in mind when studying the model that the borders to these circles are very porous; relationships can transition from one circle to another through your own actions and those of others. Are any circles emptier than others? Is this something you want to change, and if so, how? Do you see any connections that you've not noticed before? Consider what you might do to remind yourself of the importance of these relationships in your life.

Interpersonal strategies 149

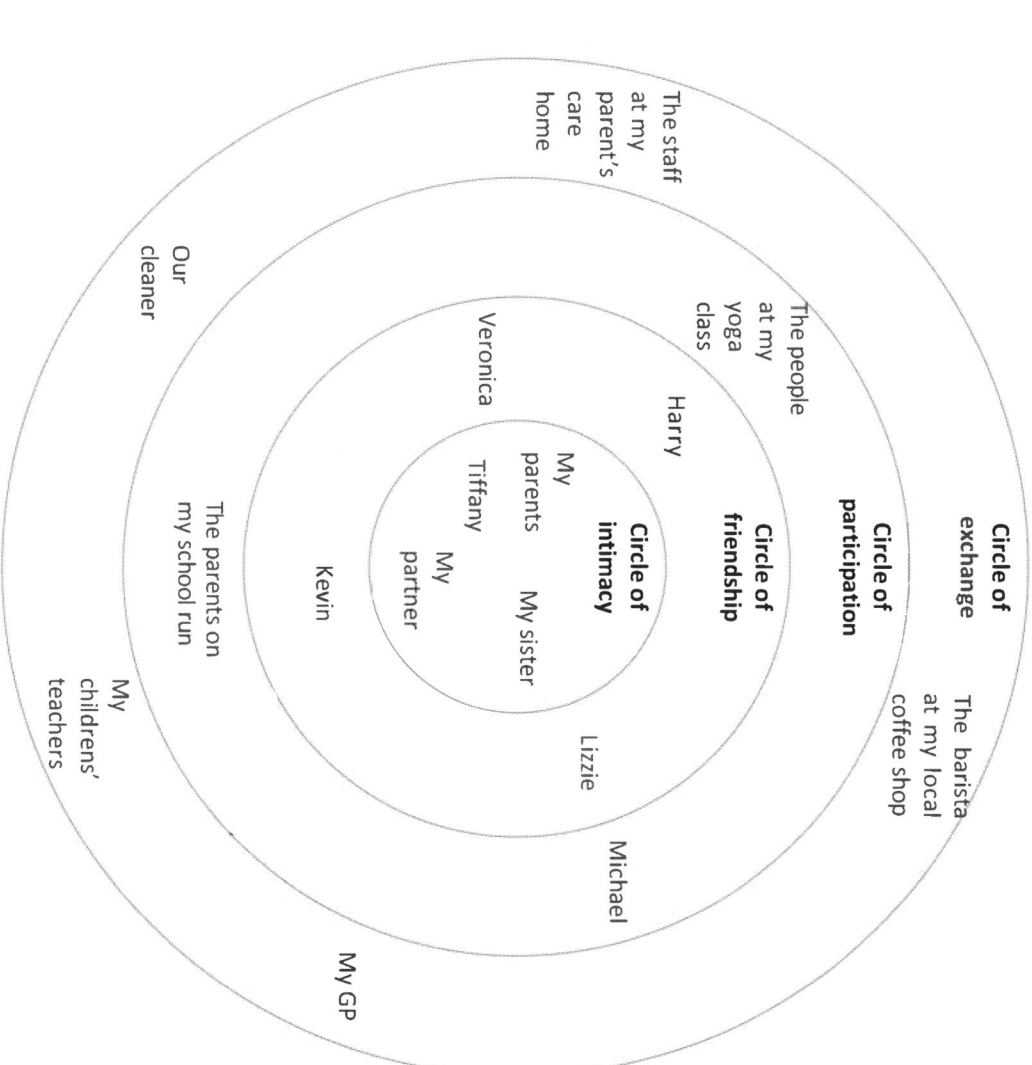

Circle of Contact

7.6 Responsibility Pie

Greenberger, D. & Padesky, C.A. (1995). *Mind over mood: A cognitive therapy treatment manual for clients.* Guilford Press.

Purpose

A Responsibility Pie can help you acknowledge how much responsibility you have for a certain situation. When we believe that we are responsible for something, we usually spend a lot of time and energy thinking about how to resolve it. If our responsibility is actually quite small, there's not much we can do about it. If our responsibility is large, but we feel we still can't do much to change the situation, our worries may persist and the stress will accumulate over time. This can be a very frustrating situation, but it can be remedied.

You can use the Responsibility Pie to identify who is responsible for an unpleasant situation that you are in and what percentage of responsibility each protagonist should be allocated. Doing so may stop you taking the blame and feeling guilty, if that is your tendency. By making clear who is responsible, even if you don't tell anyone else, you can silence your inner critic and manage your worries more effectively. You might not be able to resolve the situation, but by understanding and acknowledging your role, you can change the effects that the situation is having on you. It may also, of course, challenge you to acknowledge your actual responsibility in the situation so you can act differently in future and change the situation.

Suitability

This model is useful if you have a habit of taking responsibility for things that are outside your control. While we may be able to influence others, we cannot be held accountable for everything they do. By recognising our actual responsibility for something, we can take steps to stop worrying so much about it. After all, if all our worrying doesn't provide any solutions, then it serves no purpose and we can put our energies towards things we can do something about.

How to use

Choose a situation that is causing you anxiety or stress. Then list on the worksheet all those who you believe have some responsibility for the situation: those who created the situation, those who are affected by it and those who will benefit if the situation is resolved. They can be people, organisations or even governments. You will see on the worksheet that you have been automatically added at the bottom of the list. Then give each protagonist a responsibility score from 0–100%, based on how much you believe they are responsible for the situation. Finish by scoring yourself. In total, the scores should add up to 100%.

Write the scores on the pie. It can be helpful to see a graphic representation of how you have apportioned the responsibility. One of two things should be clear now: either you have given yourself a small slice of the pie and now need to ask yourself why you are exerting so much worry and time on something that you have such a small influence over; or you have given yourself a large slice of the pie and so should start to consider why, when you have so much responsibility, you have such little power to resolve the situation. If, in fact, you do have some means to change it, consider using SMART Goals (Chapter 2, p.32) to figure out how you can implement those changes in a specific and realistic manner.

Interpersonal strategies 151

Situation
My son not being at the top of his class

My son	40%
His teachers	20%
My partner	10%
His tutor	20%
His school friends	5%
Myself	15 %
Total	100 %

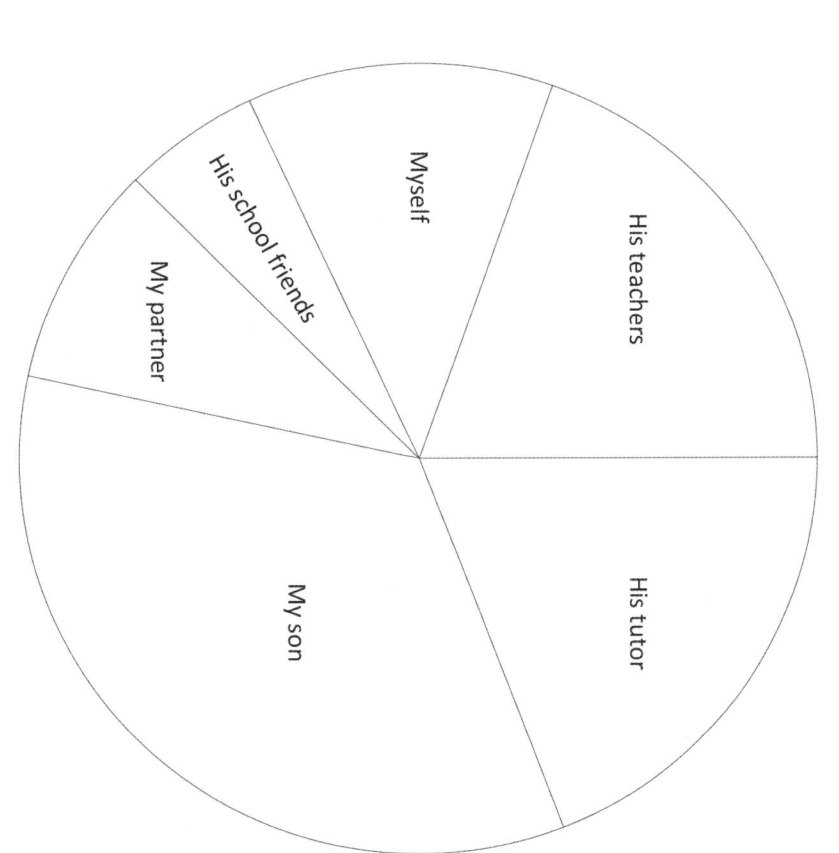

Responsibility Pie

7.7 Cycle of Abuse

Walker, L.E. (1989). Psychology and violence against women. *American Psychologist, 44*(4), 695–702.

Purpose

When you are recovering from an abusive relationship, it can be helpful to understand some of the recurring patterns that characterised the relationship. Cycle of Abuse is a way of looking at relationships that follow a pattern of bursts of explosive incidents, followed by apologies, followed by a steady increase in tension before another explosion. When this is the underlying dynamic in a relationship, we begin to tell ourselves stories about why such things are happening to us. Often these stories attribute responsibility to us: we did something to deserve the violence. These stories are distortions deriving from the stress we were under. No one deserves to be beaten up or psychologically tormented. Nevertheless, this unravelling can be difficult. Cycle of Abuse is designed to reduce our misplaced sense of guilt. If we can see the abusive relationship as inherently flawed, we will not be so quick to blame ourselves for its failure.

Suitability

Abuse can sometimes be difficult to recognise when it is not constant but follows a cycle of violence, reprieve, escalation and back to violence. Cycle of Abuse can highlight this pattern. If you currently believe you are in an abusive relationship, you should seek additional support to ensure that you are safe from harm. Once you have that security, consider using this model to reflect on your past relationship to better understand how abuse can be perpetuated.

How to use

Begin by recording abusive incidents that have occurred in a past relationship. These can include verbal, physical, sexual or financial abuse. Continue by exploring what would normally happen after these incidents. Would there be an apology? Would the abuser go out of their way to show you how much they cared for you? This is sometimes referred to as the 'honeymoon' phase, where an individual will attempt to absolve themselves of past crimes by over-compensating with kindness and gestures of affection. Use the model to write down any specific behaviours or speeches that you remember them doing.

Unfortunately, the reprieve is usually short lived, and after an abuser believes that they have been forgiven, the tension will slowly begin to accumulate again. Think back and consider what signs allowed you to see that tension was building up in your household. Arguments, name-calling and displays of aggression can all be counted as evidence that everything was not as it should be. Be wary of blaming yourself for this tension. It is easy to internalise the voice of your abuser and begin to believe the things that are said of you, to the point where you take responsibility for the abuse you are receiving.

When you have completed the model, focus your attention on the centre and consider why the word 'denial' is written there. Denial can touch on all the stages of the cycle and it is worth investigating who might have been in denial and, if they were, what it was that they were denying exactly. Consider this and any other thoughts that are brought to the surface.

Interpersonal strategies 153

Cycle of Abuse

Tension building

They get angry at me over the smallest things

They are irritable with the children

They spend less time at home

They begin to criticise my performance/appearance/attitude

DENIAL

Honeymoon

They help out with household chores and looking after the kids

They buy me presents

They are more responsive to my needs

They are apologetic about the past if it ever comes up

Incident

They throw something across the room

They yell at me

They call the police and say that I have been acting violently

They threaten to hurt me and my family

Chapter 8. Relapse prevention

Introduction

Hopefully, if you have been using some of the models in the preceding chapters, you will by now have begun to see some changes in how you manage problem situations in your life. Perhaps your difficulties are not as intense as they were, or you now feel more confident to use the models and coping devices you have learned here. Ideally, you should now have an understanding of what improves your mental health and wellbeing and your own role and potential for maintaining your emotional and behavioural equilibrium.

This chapter is concerned partly with refreshing your memory about these lessons and partly with equipping you to deal with possible relapses. Simply integrating a model into your daily life is no guarantee that you will never have a panic attack or depressive episode again. Life is stressful; all we can do is try to ensure the fluctuations stay within manageable boundaries and do not overwhelm us.

When looking back at the progress you have made, it can be helpful to write down what you have noticed has changed in your life. The Improvement and Impact Reflection worksheet (p.156) is where you can record what is different now and how it might connect with any new outlooks or behaviours you have adopted. If you are feeling better, it is always worth making the effort to understand why that might be and giving yourself a pat on the back if it's merited. The small changes we make in how we see and behave in the world can have a much bigger impact than we think, often because it ripples out to the people around us. If we are able to identify these changes, we are more likely to notice if they begin to fade away and we are better able to stop that happening. New Coping Devices Reflection (p.158) encourages you to look at the review and coping techniques you have learned and ensure they remain present in your mind.

While celebrating your successes, it is important not to have too high an expectation of yourself to maintain them. If you think that you have banished your depression, your angry outbursts or your moments of panic forever, you will be all the more devastated if they come back. The Progress not Perfection Charts (p.160) encourage you to recognise the progress you have made and avoid the tyranny of perfectionism. The worksheet allows you to review the progress you have made in dealing with your problematic thoughts and behaviours without seeing them as entirely eradicated forever.

If you do start to fall back into old habits, Early Warning Signs (p.162) can help you recognise when you are having difficulties again. The models in this book can be referred back to at any time if the need recurs. That is the nature of self-improvement: it is continuous (or should be), and it never ends. Rather, it evolves, just as you do as a person.

If a relapse occurs, Action Plan (p.164) will help you write up your own, personalised strategy, drawing on the techniques in this book that you have found work well for you. Having a plan to hand when things start to go wrong or a crisis strikes makes it easier to handle whatever comes your way.

Then we come to Future Plans (p.166). I suggest you create two: one that concerns your long-term life goals and consolidates everything you have learnt here, and another that anticipates that there will be a few bumps in the road and you will need some resources to ensure you stay on course. This is a very practical model that allows you to look towards the future with one eye on the past.

With the other chapters, you could pick and choose the models that you completed in each section. With this chapter, I recommend that you complete all the models here – this will be your relapse plan, to take with you on your journey forward. You should be able to find something in all the models in this chapter that speaks to you and can help you along the way. This is an opportunity to review, reflect and congratulate yourself on the progress that you have made so far.

8.1 Improvement and Impact Reflection

Marlatt, G.A. & Donovan, D.M. (2005). *Relapse prevention: Maintenance strategies in the treatment of addictive behaviours*. Guilford Press.

Purpose

When learning new skills and techniques that sustain your mental health and wellbeing, it is worth assessing their impact when you start to see measurable improvement in how you feel. It can be very rewarding to see how small changes have had a significant impact on how you deal with others, how you resolve problems and what you do to manage your mood. By taking the time to look back at what you have accomplished, you can see what has worked and what hasn't and be better prepared to overcome future obstacles with the tools that you have found helpful.

Suitability

Improvement and Impact Reflection provides a means for you to summarise the benefits of the models you have completed so that you can more easily see how different aspects of your life have improved. Therapeutic interventions often have a gradual impact on your perceptions and behaviours, which can make it all the more important to periodically review your progress and recognise your own work towards this.

How to use

Reflect on what has changed in your life since you decided to start resolving your issues. Look for physical changes and also for changes in how you look at the world and relationships since you started this work. Look at each area on the worksheet – work/studies/contribution, family, home life, friendships/relationships, social life – and explore the impact of your new thinking and behaviour in each section. There will be some overlap between them: for instance, you might find that friendships and social life blend into one another. If this is the case, consider what this tells you about the nature of each and their interconnection, and what might happen if one were to be neglected.

When completing this worksheet, you should ideally see it as part celebration of what you have achieved and part analysis of the results of your efforts. It is common for people to minimise how much they contribute to their own suffering through unhealthy coping behaviours and unhelpful thinking patterns. In the same way, when things go right and start to improve, some people have a tendency to attribute the changes to luck or to the interventions of others. This minimises the significance of our own efforts and perpetuates a sense of helplessness. When you are filling in this worksheet, be sure to emphasise what you personally have done to improve your situation.

Improvement and Impact Reflection

Work/studies/contribution
I have noticed that I am dreading going to work less. I no longer want to stay in bed in the morning. My sleep has improved and this has an impact on my energy levels. Where before I would get tired at work in the afternoon, I am now more able to stay productive for the whole day. I think this has improved my relationships at work as I am not so short-tempered as before

Family
Since talking with my family about delegating jobs around the house, I am under less stress. I am worried that it will be hard to maintain, though, and that I will have to chase and nag them to make sure they keep to the rota. I think they see that they need to be more responsible and I need to be less controlling

Home life
One of my goals was to find the energy to do more at home and to re-engage with the hobbies that I used to do after work, like going for a swim and sewing. I have found that finding the time to do things for myself has really decreased my stress levels, but that I need to be aware that I don't take it for granted and skip those activities when I am tired

Friendships/relationships
I have been making a more concentrated attempt to spend more time with my friends, even if that just means a call every now and again. I always leave those interactions feeling refreshed and in a better mood. I think having that support network outside my family is quite useful as there are some things I can't discuss with my family that I can with friends

Social life
My social life has improved somewhat as I am more willing now to prioritise that part of my life, even if it means that my attention can't be on work or my family to the same extent. The rationale that I need to help myself in order to help others has had a big impact on how I see things like going for a drink with colleagues or going to my sports club

8.2 New Coping Devices Reflection

Wells, A. (1997). *Cognitive therapy of anxiety disorders: A practice manual and conceptual guide.* John Wiley & Sons.

Purpose

Improving and maintaining healthy coping devices is essential to seeing consistent progress. When you reflect on what you have learned in this book, pay attention to the behaviours and techniques you have developed that either reduce stress or anxiety or lift your mood. These are often the first things you can do to manage your mood better on your own, so they are a crucial component in independent learning and in becoming your own therapist.

New Coping Devices Reflection allows you to quickly assess the coping devices you have found helpful and the strategies that help you implement them. There will, hopefully, be some variety in the list; it's good to have a breadth of choice as it allows you some flexibility to adapt the techniques you use to changing circumstances.

Suitability

This model is useful for people who want to review the new coping devices they have learned. It can be of particular use if you previously had a number of unhealthy coping devices and have been slowly replacing them with healthier alternatives. Similarly, if you were experiencing a lot of stress and had little time for yourself, this model can remind you of the importance of taking the time to focus on your own health and maintain these coping devices in your daily routine.

How to use

First, consider which therapeutic worksheets in this book have been particularly relevant and useful to you. It may be that only a few of the models speak to your needs and offer you relevant guidance and support. List them on this worksheet. Then list any non-therapeutic coping techniques that have been helpful. These might be things that you used to do but stopped when your problems intensified. Or they might be new activities that you have enjoyed and give you a sense of achievement. Exercise, meditation, spending time with friends and family would all fall under this category.

Maintaining a combination of the therapeutic and non-therapeutic is, in my view, the best strategy moving forward. However, you may find that, as time progresses and your ability to manage stresses in your life improves, you use the non-therapeutic coping strategies more often and you have less need for the models in this book.

But before you reach that point, it is worth using this worksheet to record what you can do to ensure that your coping techniques remain present in your life. You may want to start using a diary as a continual record. There will be moments when you slip and stumble, but by applying the coping devices you have learned and practised here, you can reduce how far you fall and picking yourself up will be all the easier.

New Coping Devices Reflection

What therapeutic skills/exercises have proven helpful?

Cognitive Maintenance Model

Worry Diary

Worry Tree

Responsibility Pie

What non-therapeutic activities have proven helpful?

Jogging

Baking

Finding time for friends

Helping my daughter with her homework

Meditation

What has helped me put these skills and activities into practice?

Keeping a schedule

Setting reminders and alarms on my phone

Getting my partner Involved with what I am doing and how they can help

Being kinder to myself when I make mistakes

8.3 Progress not Perfection Charts

Shafran, R., Egan, S. & Wade, T. (2018). *Overcoming perfectionism: A self-help guide using cognitive behavioural techniques*. Robinson.

Purpose

Progress not Perfection Charts can be used to measure your progress and see what has improved in your life since you first set out to make changes. However, they also clarify what progress looks like by inviting you to reflect on what perfection might be. Don't regard this as a goal-setting exercise; on the contrary, its purpose is to help you to realise what is attainable and what might always be impossible to achieve.

While we can surround ourselves with a strong support system and adopt healthy coping strategies, there is nothing we can do to guarantee that we won't face challenges that test us again in similar ways. Rather than trying to keep yourself safe and protected from such adversities, it is far better to build confidence in the models you have successfully used and know you can use them again if needed.

Suitability

When striving to improve your health, it is helpful to see your goals in terms of progress, not perfection. Perfection is impossible to achieve. By setting a standard so high, you set yourself up to fail. But if you track your progress and see incremental change, you can see that you are moving in the right direction. Use the Progress not Perfection Charts to remind yourself of the progress you have made on each of your problems. Anyone will benefit from using this model, but people with perfectionist traits will derive additional benefit from understanding that a more realistic aim is to make progress in your ability to manage the intensity and resulting impacts of your problem thoughts and behaviours, not eradicate them.

How to use

Start by listing on the worksheet some of the problems that you have been dealing with in recent weeks. You might want to phrase them in quite general terms, such as worrying too much or feeling depressed in the evenings, or you might want to be more specific and focus on particular physical symptoms that you have been experiencing or practical challenges that you have been facing. Then write down what perfection would look like for each issue – what would it look like if that problem was entirely resolved? If you worry too much, perhaps perfection would look like never worrying again. You may start to see immediately that some of these perfection targets are impossible to achieve, but write them down anyway.

Now record how you felt at the start with each problem. How terrible was it? Describe this briefly but in clear detail. Next, write down the progress you have made since your problem became apparent. This is where you look back at the steps you have taken so that you can appreciate how far you have come. Instead of focusing on perfection, focus on the distance between where you used to be and where you are now. If you were able to make that sort of progress in the past, consider what you might be able to do in the future.

Progress not Perfection Charts

Issue	'Perfection'	Where I started	Progress
Bursting into tears over small things	Complete control of my emotional reactions	On days where I felt very low, the smallest thing might set me off	Though I still get emotional, I haven't cried at all in the last few weeks

Issue	'Perfection'	Where I started	Progress
Feeling others are constantly judging my performance	Being confident in everything that I do	I would avoid saying much in public or in groups	I still feel that others might be judging me, but I now look for evidence of this

Issue	'Perfection'	Where I started	Progress
Getting into arguments with my mother	Never getting into arguments with her	We would argue on a daily basis and it would often escalate to shouting	We still argue a few times a week, but I am able to prevent it from getting out of control

Issue	'Perfection'	Where I started	Progress

Issue	'Perfection'	Where I started	Progress

8.4 Early Warning Signs

Marlatt, G.A. & Donovan, D.M. (2005). *Relapse prevention: Maintenance strategies in the treatment of addictive behaviours*. Guilford Press.

Purpose

Intense emotional states can sometimes occur suddenly and without warning. However, often there are signs before a crisis that things are not as they should be. If you can recognise these warning signs, you may be able to act early to prevent the situation escalating further. This model requires you to reflect on your past and identify physical symptoms, emotional episodes or particular behaviours that usually emerge and escalate when things are starting to go seriously awry. Once you have an understanding of these early warning signs, you can devise and implement an Action Plan (p.164) so you don't lose the progress you have made here.

Suitability

Similar to many models in this chapter, the intention behind Early Warning Signs is to prepare you for times when you need to draw on the techniques learnt here and reapply them in future situations. People who tend to have quite intense emotional episodes that take a significant length of time to recover from may find this model particularly helpful.

How to use

Write down the warnings signs that suggest that things aren't going so well. These might include poor sleep, migraines, irritability, or spontaneous crying. Many warning signs are quite personal, but they will all suggest that your equilibrium has been thrown off balance in some way and needs to be regained. Warning signs do not necessarily have to be emotional or physical states. They can also include thinking patterns that you notice yourself falling into more and more often. By looking ahead you can prepare yourself for the possibility of emotional distress and check that you have the tools to deal with the challenges likely to be coming your way. But I want to emphasise that this model is not an invitation to worry excessively about hypothetical fears and doubts. Early Warning Signs should simply serve as a means to identify and record these signs so you can act to resolve them before they become uncontrollable.

Early Warning Signs

Early warning sign

An early warning sign of things going back to how they were would be if my sleep started to suffer again and I was only getting 5–6 hours a night

Early warning sign

When I start cancelling plans to see friends and spend more time alone in my house

Early warning sign

When I find myself ruminating about the past and things that I can't change

Early warning sign

Putting off important tasks and failing to meet deadlines

8.5 Action Plan

Nezu, A.M., Maguth Nezu, C. & D'Zurilla, T.J. (2013). *Problem-solving therapy: A treatment manual.* Springer Publishing Co.

Purpose

An Action Plan is a blueprint for what to do in an emergency. Sometimes taking two steps forward will involve taking one step back. Instead of becoming disheartened or losing faith in your accomplishments, use any setbacks as opportunities to refine the skills that you have been developing here. But it is best to complete this model when you are feeling confident in your abilities. If in the future that confidence fails you, you will not have to remember what works or start from scratch; you can simply follow your own advice here.

Suitability

Action Plan is a very necessary part of your self-support package. Setbacks are natural and by preparing for them in advance you will be better able to deal with any future obstacles and reduce the likelihood that those setbacks will overwhelm you. Action Plan encourages you to think through and write down the steps you need to take in a crisis, what you have learned about your triggers, the techniques and strategies you know work for you and how you will know they are working for you again now.

How to use

Begin by listing your triggers on the worksheet. Your triggers might be specific social interactions, significant life events, news stories, times of the year, a flare-up of a health condition and so on. Being able to identify these triggers can make you more aware of the effect that they have on you, not so you can avoid them but so you can redirect your attention elsewhere. The difference between these two strategies is crucial. Many stressful things simply cannot be avoided, but when they befall you, you do have control over how much attention you give them. Remember, excessive attention is responsible for overwhelming anxiety as well as the ruminating that we do when we feel depressed. So you need to list on this model the redirection strategies that you can deploy when triggers likely to lead to stress reactions occur.

Then list ways you can problem-solve the situation. These can be more complex than simply focusing your attention on something other than the situation; they also include using therapeutic tools and strategies that have worked well for you in the past and may again in the future – so list them here. List the models in this book that you have found helpful.

When thinking about how to go about applying these methods, use the SMART Goals model (Chapter 2, p.32) to make your intentions specific, measurable, achievable, relevant and time sensitive. This can help with procrastination and give you clear targets to aim for.

Finally, complete the worksheet by stating clearly how you will know that you have successfully applied your plan. Success might be indicated by a change in your behaviour or in how your body feels, or changes in your relationships with others, or you no longer performing the ritual actions that you used to use to help you feel safe.

Action Plan

What are my triggers?	Too much work Poor sleep Money worries Dealing with bureaucracy
How can I redirect my attention?	Focus on my exercise goals Breathing exercises Watch TV in the evenings Speak to my partner about something unrelated
What tools can I use to resolve the situation?	Progressive Muscle Relaxation Stress Quadrant Problematic Behaviour Diary Friendship network
How do I keep it SMART?	Break up the problem into small, manageable goals Keep track of everything that I do so I can measure progress Set myself targets to reach in the short term
How will I know if what I am trying is working?	I will see an improvement in my interactions with others I will not feel so emotionally drained I will sleep better I will have more energy in the day to do things I enjoy

8.6 Future Plans

Stanley, B. & Brown, G.K. (2012). Safety planning intervention: A brief intervention to mitigate suicide risk. *Cognitive and Behavioral Practice*, *19*(2), 256–264.

Purpose

The purpose of Future Plans is to help you look to the future with an idea of what to expect next. As such, it provides a space to discuss how you will build on your existing knowledge and skills and supplement them with further plans and goals. These plans will ensure that, if there is a setback, you will be able to manage it more effectively. By writing down your plans, you are in a way making a pledge to take with you what you have learned here on the next stages of your journey.

Suitability

This model is designed to ensure that you take into the future what you have learnt from using this book. It is helpful to see how what you have achieved so far has laid the foundations for your next steps. This is both constructive, in the sense that you build on what you have learned, and preventive, in ensuring that, if you have any setbacks, you will know how to handle them. Future Plans also serves to remind you that you are not alone. Acknowledging your support system should give you confidence to venture forth knowing that, if you trip, there are people around you to help pick you up.

How to use

First, explore how you can build on everything that you have learned from working through this book. How can you continue the learning process on your own? If you struggle to imagine how you can build on what you have developed, think about your long-term goals and where you see yourself in a year or 10 years' time. How can you get there with the techniques and coping devices you have? Do they need further work? If so, consider further practice of these models, reading more psychology books and exposing yourself to new challenges. The list of options is potentially endless.

Then take time to reflect on how you would deal with setbacks. What might you do? None of us is free from the possibility that some life event may change things for the worse. If this were to happen, you would not be powerless to change things back. The work you have done up to now is a testament to your ability to overcome challenges. It is important to remember this, especially when you are feeling down and unmotivated.

Were that to happen, be sure not just to rely on your abilities; reach out to your wider support system, which might include family, friends, community and activity groups and mental health organisations. List the people you can trust to provide you with support and keep the completed worksheet somewhere safe to remind you when you need it.

Future Plans

How do I build on what I have learned?

I will start by printing out copies of the therapeutic exercises and putting them in a folder so I have access to them whenever I might need them in the future. I will build on the goals that I have achieved in the past few weeks by adding more long-term goals – for example, by imagining where I want to be in 10 years' time and working backwards from there. I will start looking for a new job that will be more rewarding and I will use the strategies that I have learned here to deal with any rejection that I might face in that process

How do I deal with setbacks?

I will remember that setbacks are normal; that progress is not a straight line upwards. I can practise the CBT strategies that I have learned and implement them to manage aspects of my life that I am struggling with

Who can I contact for additional support?

My partner

My GP

My therapist

My online peer support group

Further support and resources

NHS therapy services

For people living in England (those in Scotland, Wales and Northern Ireland have equivalent but different systems), the main source of primary care counselling for people experiencing mental distress is the Improving Access to Psychological Therapies (IAPT) programme. IAPT is an NHS primary care programme that offers evidence-based talking therapies to adults with a range of mental health difficulties. The treatment is primarily cognitive-behavioural therapy (CBT) or self-help based on CBT principles, although some local services offer a wider choice of therapies, and is delivered through telephone, digital, one-to-one and group formats. There is also an IAPT programme for children and young people, but this is integrated within the wider spcialist Child and Adolescent Mental Health Services (CAMHS) for that age group.

In some areas you can refer yourself to IAPT; in others, you need to get your GP to do so. IAPT services can also link you to other support services in your area and refer you to secondary care if you need more help.

As this is an NHS service, IAPT therapy is free and confidential. Seek out their support first, unless you already have a clear idea of what you need. Go to **www.nhs.uk** and search for **IAPT** to find local services.

As above, children and young people can access NHS counselling through their local CAMHS.

For people with more severe mental health difficulties, there is a limited NHS secondary care psychology service offering psychological therapies, which is accessed via initial GP referral or referral through primary mental health services.

Counselling and psychotherapy

If you are willing to pay, there is a huge number of counsellors and psychotherapists working privately, or in small partnerships, across the UK, and larger, independent-sector agencies. There are also a few charities (local and national) that offer free or low-cost counselling and therapy. Generally, if you search online for 'low-cost counselling' in your area, you will find them, or ask your local Citizens Advice Bureau. To find a private therapist, I suggest you consult the websites of the main professional bodies that register or represent them. They have online directories that list their practising members by area and speciality:

Black, African and Asian Therapy Network (BAATN)
www.baatn.org.uk

British Association for Counselling and Psychotherapy (BACP)
www.bacp.co.uk

British Association of Behavioural and Cognitive Psychotherapists (BABCP)
www.babcp.com

National Counselling Society (NCS)
https://nationalcounsellingsociety.org

UK Council for Psychotherapy (UKCP)
www.psychotherapy.org.uk

Voluntary sector support and information

In addition, there are voluntary sector groups that provide information, advice and sometimes specialist counselling for particular groups and specialist needs:

The Arbours Association
www.arboursassociation.org

Institute of Family Therapy
www.ift.org.uk

Marriage Care
www.marriagecare.org.uk

Mind
www.mind.org.uk

Relate (relationship difficulties)
www.relate.org.uk

Children and young people

Childline
Telephone: 0800 1111
www.childline.org.uk

NSPCC (children's welfare)
Telephone: 0808 800 5000
www.nspcc.org.uk

Young Minds (children and young people)
www.youngminds.org.uk

Crisis helplines

Calm (male suicide support)
Telephone: 0800 58 58 58
www.thecalmzone.net

Samaritans
Telephone: 116 123
www.samaritans.org

Supportline (for mental health issues across all ages)
Telephone: 01708 765200
www.supportline.org.uk

Specialist mental health support

Action on Postpartum Psychosis
Telephone: 020 33229900
www.app-network.org

Anxiety UK
Telephone: 03444 775 774
www.anxietyuk.org.uk

Beat (eating disorder support)
Telephone: 0808 801 0677
www.beateatingdisorders.org.uk

Depression UK
www.depressionuk.org

Grassroots (suicide prevention and awareness service)
Telephone: 01273 675764
www.prevent-suicide.org.uk

Hearing Voices Network
www.hearing-voices.org

Mencap (support for people with learning disabilities and their family and carers)
Telephone: 0808 808 1111
www.mencap.org.uk

National Autistic Society
Telephone: 0808 800 4104
www.autism.org.uk

National Self-Harm Network (NSHN)
www.nshn.co.uk

No Panic
Telephone: 0808 8080545
www.nopanic.org.uk

OCD Action
Telephone: 0845 390 6232
www.ocdaction.org.uk

Overeaters Anonymous
Telephone: 07798 587802
www.oagb.org.uk

PTSD Resolution (for UK armed forces veterans)
Telephone: 0300 302 0551
www.ptsdresolution.org

Self-Injury Support
Telephone: 0808 800 8088
www.selfinjurysupport.org.uk

Talk ED
www.talk-ed.org.uk

Triumph over Phobia
Telephone: 01225 571740
www.topuk.org

Mental health general

For more information about mental health, access to services, legal issues and so on:

Mind
Telephone: 0300 123 3393
www.mind.org.uk

NHS Choices
Telephone: 111
www.nhs.uk

Rethink
Telephone: 0300 5000 927
www.rethink.org

Violence and abuse

Forced Marriage Unit
Telephone: 01642 683 045
www.haloproject.org.uk

Galop (for victims of LGBTQI+ assault)
Telephone: 020 7704 2040
www.galop.org.uk

NAPAC (sexual abuse in childhood)
Telephone: 0808 801 0331
www.napac.org.uk

Rape Crisis
Telephone: 0808 802 9999
www.rapecrisis.org.uk

Refuge (safe housing for women experiencing domestic abuse)
Telephone: 0808 2000 247
www.refuge.org.uk

Respect (help for domestic violence perpetrators)
Telephone: 0808 8024040
www.respectphoneline.org.uk

Woman's Trust (for women experiencing domestic violence)
Telephone: 020 7034 0303
www.womanstrust.org.uk

Women and Girls Network
Telephone: 0808 801 0660
www.wgn.org.uk

Addiction support

1NE Teens (for children whose parents or carers have addiction issues)
Telephone: 020 8220 0132
www.1ne.org.uk/services/ne-teens

Adfam (support for families affected by drug or alcohol abuse)
Telephone: 020 3817 9410
www.adfam.org.uk

Alcoholics Anonymous
Telephone: 0800 9177 650
www.alcoholics-anonymous.org.uk

Drink Aware
Telephone: 020 7766 9900
www.drinkaware.co.uk

Frank (drug addiction support)
Telephone: 0300 1236600
www.talktofrank.com

Gamblers Anonymous
Telephone: 0330 094 0322
www.gamblersanonymous.org.uk

Gamcare
Telephone: 0808 802 0133
www.gamcare.org.uk

Taking Action on Addiction
Telephone: 0300 330 0659
www.actiononaddiction.org.uk

Well Aware
Telephone: 0300 123 1110
www.wellaware.org.uk

Further support and resources 173

Bereavement support
Bereavement Advice Centre
Telephone: 0800 634 9494
www.bereavementadvice.org

Child Bereavement UK (support after the death of a child)
Telephone: 0800 02 888 40
www.childbereavementuk.org

Child Death Helpline
Telephone: 0800 282 986
Website: www.childdeathhelpline.org.uk

Compassionate Friends (peer support for the bereaved)
Telephone: 0345 123 2304
www.tcf.org.uk

Cruse Bereavement Support
Telephone: 0808 808 1677
www.cruse.org.uk

Survivors of Bereavement by Suicide
Telephone: 0300 111 5065
www.uksobs.org

Winston's Wish (support for bereaved children)
Telephone: 08088 020 021
www.winstonswish.org

Carers
Carers Trust
Telephone: 0300 772 9600
www.carers.org

Carers UK
Telephone: 020 7378 4999
www.carersuk.org

Employment and mental health
ACAS (advice and information concerning employment and legal rights)
Telephone: 0300 123 1100
www.acas.org.uk

BITC (business network for mental health promotion in the workplace)
Telephone: 020 7566 8650
www.bitc.org.uk

Mental Health at Work (information for employers to support employees with mental health issues)
www.mentalhealthatwork.org.uk

Richmond Fellowship (employment and housing support)
Telephone: 020 7697 3300
www.richmondfellowship.org.uk

Older Adults

Age UK
Telephone: 0800 678 1602
www.ageuk.org.uk

Alzheimer's Society
Telephone: 0333 150 3456
www.alzheimers.org.uk

Dementia UK
Telephone: 0800 888 6678
www.dementiauk.org

Reengage (recreational activities for older adults)
Telephone: 0800 716543
www.reengage.org.uk

The Silverline
Telephone: 0800 470 8090
www.thesilverline.org.uk

U3A (educational courses for older adults)
Telephone: 020 8466 6139
www.u3a.org.uk

Housing

Christians Against Poverty (debt, unemployment and housing support)
Telephone: 0800 328 0006
www.capuk.org

Micro Rainbow (LGBTQI+ housing, employment, training and education)
Telephone: 020 3559 6490
www.microrainbow.org

Salvation Army
Telephone: 020 7367 4800
www.salvationarmy.org.uk

Shelter (support for homeless people)
Telephone: 0808 800 4444
www.shelter.org.uk

SHP (support for those experiencing homelessness)
Telephone: 0204 509 8300
www.shp.org.uk

Stonewall Housing (LGBTQI+ housing support)
Telephone: 020 7359 5767
https://stonewallhousing.org

Refugee support

Freedom from Torture (counselling and support for torture survivors)
020 7697 7777
www.freedomfromtorture.org

Helen Bamber Foundation (for refugees and asylum seekers who have experienced violence and abuse)
Telephone: 0203 058 2020
www.helenbamber.org

Mental Health and Human Rights Info (database of helpful sources concerning mental health in war/conflict areas)
www.hhri.org

Micro Rainbow (LGBTQI+ refugees)
Telephone: 020 3559 6490
www.microrainbow.org

Refugee Action
Telephone: 07753 325364
www.refugee-action.org.uk

Refugee Council
Telephone: 0808 196 7272
www.refugeecouncil.org.uk

Online counselling/peer support

Kooth
www.kooth.com

Qwell
www.qwell.io

Togetherall (online community for mental health support)
https://togetherall.com/en-gb

Self-help apps

These are just some of many on the market. Inclusion here is not a recommendation.

Beat Panic
www.au.reachout.com/tools-and- apps/beat-panic

Be Mindful (mindfulness-based cognitive therapy)
www.bemindfulonline.com

Calm Harm (self-harm management)
www.calmharm.co.uk

Catch It (CBT-based diary for mood management)
www.liverpool.ac.uk/it/app-directory/catch-it/

Chill Panda (relaxation and worry management)
www.chillpanda.co.uk

Companion (online mental health workshops for employees)
www.companionapproach.com

DistrACT (advice and information about self-harm and suicide prevention)
www.expertselfcare.com/health-apps/distract

Headspace (mindfulness and meditation)
www.headspace.com

ieso (online courses with text-based communication with therapists)
www.iesohealth.com/en-gb

Living Life to the Full (online courses for low mood, stress and resilience)
www.llttf.com

SilverCloud (CBT-based digital therapy)
www.silvercloudhealth.com/uk

Sleepstation (sleep management tool)
www.sleepstation.org.uk

Sleepio (sleep management)
Website: www.sleepio.com

Stay Alive (suicide prevention)
www.prevent-suicide.org.uk/find-help-now/stay-alive-app

Student Health App (health information for students)
www.expertselfcare.com/health-apps/student-health-app

tellmi
www.tellmi.help

WorryTree (strategies to deal with excessive worry)
www.worry-tree.com/worrytree-mobile-app

Further reading and CBT workbooks

Antony, M.M. & Swinson, R.P. (2008). *Shyness and social anxiety workbook: Proven, step-by-step techniques for overcoming your fear* (2nd ed.). New Harbinger Publications.

Bamber, M.R. (2011). *Overcoming your workplace stress: A CBT-based self-help guide*. Routledge.

Beck, J. (2011). *Cognitive behavior therapy: Basics and beyond* (2nd ed.). Guilford Press.

Burns, D. D. (2020). *The feeling good handbook: The groundbreaking program with powerful new techniques and step-by-step exercises to overcome depression, conquer anxiety, and enjoy greater intimacy*. Plume.

Christensen, H., & Griffiths, K. (2011). *The mood gym: Overcoming depression with CBT and other effective therapies.* Vermilion.

Edelman, S. (2007). *Change your thinking: Overcome stress, anxiety, and depression, and improve your life with CBT*. Da Capo Lifelong Books.

Ellis, A., Harper, R.A. & Powers, M. (1975). *A guide to rational living.* Wilshire Book Company.

Gilbert, P. (2019). *The compassionate mind*. Robinson.

Greenberger, D., Padesky, C.A. & Beck, A.T. (2015). *Mind over mood* (2nd ed.). Guilford Press

Hayes, S.C. & Smith, S. (2005). *Get out of your mind and into your life: The new acceptance and commitment therapy*. New Harbinger Publications.

Knaus, W.J. (2021). *The cognitive behavioral workbook for anxiety: A step-by-step program*. New Harbinger Publications.

Robichaud, M. (2015). *Generalized anxiety disorder workbook: A comprehensive CBT guide for coping with uncertainty, worry, and fear.* New Harbinger Publications.

Shafran, R., Egan, S. & Wade, T. (2010). *Overcoming perfectionism.* Robinson.

Turk, D.C., & Winter, F. (2006). *The pain survival guide.* American Psychological Association.

Williams, M., Teasdale, J., Segal, Z. & Kabat-Zinn, J. (2007). *The mindful way through depression: Freeing yourself from chronic unhappiness.* Guilford Press.

Winston, S.M. (2017). *Overcoming unwanted intrusive thoughts: A CBT-based guide to getting over frightening, obsessive, or disturbing thoughts.* New Harbinger Publications.

Appendix 1: Thematic guides

Depression Template

- ABC Analysis for Behavioural Modification
- Behavioural Diary
- Identifying Activities
- Theory A/B Model
- Unhelpful Thinking Styles
- Thought-Disputing Model
- Circle of Contact
- Future Plans

Generalised Anxiety Template

- Cognitive Maintenance Model
- Reality vs Expectations
- Square Breathing Technique
- Worry Diary
- Worry Tree
- Worry Time
- Coping Cards
- New Coping Devices Reflection

Thematic guides 181

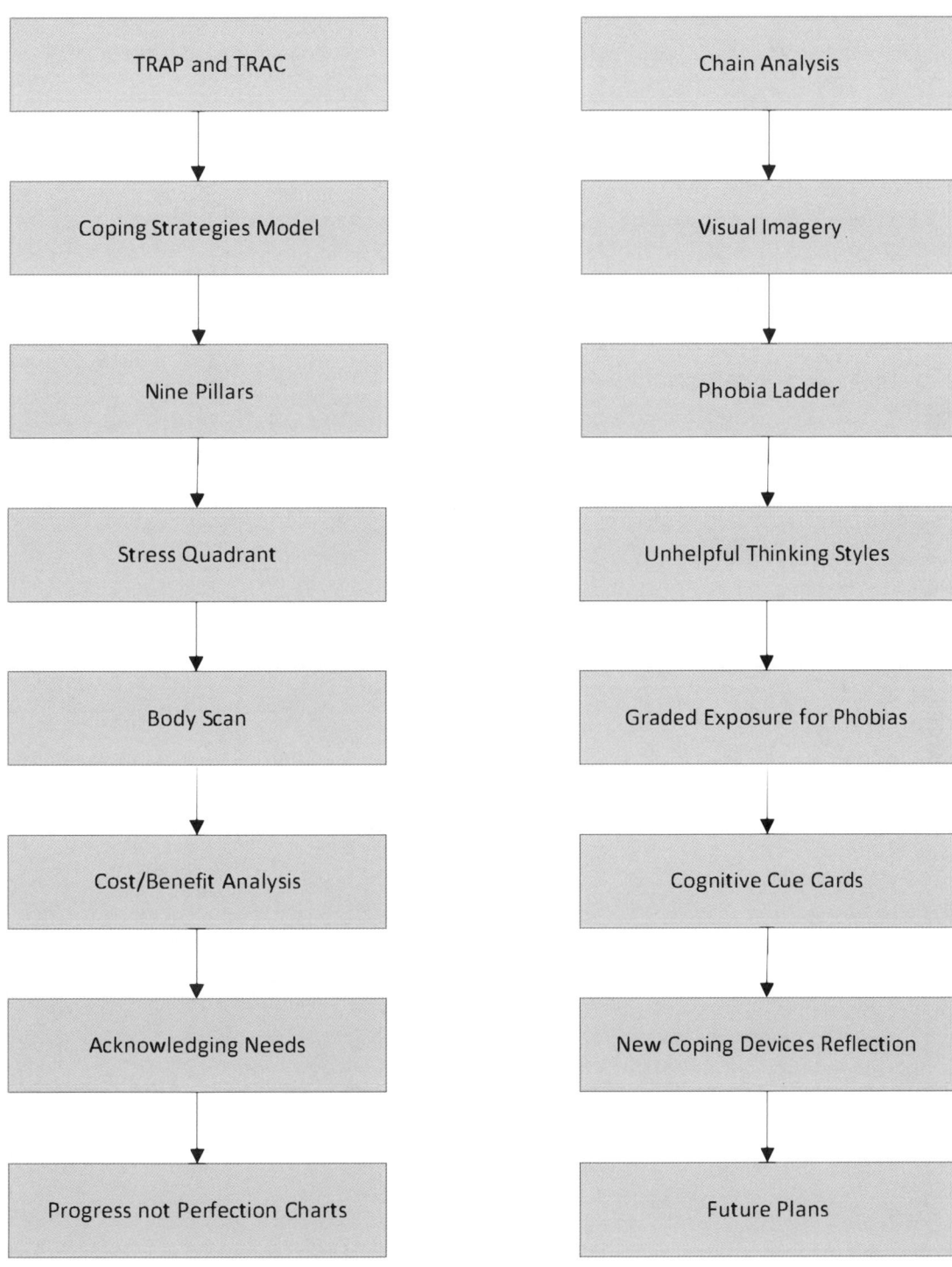

182   The CBT Companion

OCD Template

- Cognitive Model of OCD
- Progressive Muscle Relaxation
- Intrusive Thoughts Diary
- Critical Voice Record
- Cycle of Beliefs, Rules and Behaviours
- Rules into Values
- OCD Graded Exposure
- Improvement and Impact Reflection

PTSD Template

- Cognitive Model of Trauma
- SMART Goals
- Grounding
- PTSD Diary
- Core Belief Challenging
- Evidence Table for Core Beliefs
- Core Belief Experiment
- Action Plan

Appendix 2: Blank worksheets

1 Formulations

1.1	Cognitive maintenance model	185
1.2	Cognitive model of panic	186
1.3	Cognitive model of perfectionism	187
1.4	Cognitive model of obsessive-compulsive disorder	188
1.5	Cognitive model of trauma	189
1.6	Vicious flowers for health anxiety	190
1.7	TRAP and TRAC	191
1.8	Chain analysis	193
1.9	ABC analysis for behavioural modification	194
1.10	Problem development model	195
1.11	Coping strategies model	196
1.12	Biopsychosocial model of health	197

2 Goals and behavioural planning

2.1	SMART goals	198
2.2	Nine pillars	199
2.3	Sleep hygiene checklist	200
2.4	Reality vs expectations	201
2.5	Stress quadrant	202
2.6	Phobia ladder	203
2.7	Behavioural diary	204
2.8	Identifying activities	205
2.9	Alternative solutions model	206
2.10	Exploring values	207
2.11	The value compass	208

3 Relaxation

3.1	Square breathing technique	209
3.2	Visual imagery	210
3.3	Progressive muscle relaxation	211
3.4	Body scan	212
3.5	Mundane task focusing	213
3.6	Grounding	214

4 Diary keeping

4.1	Worry diary	215
4.2	Problematic behaviour diary	216
4.3	Relaxation diary	217
4.4	Food journal	218
4.5	Panic diary	219
4.6	Health anxiety thought record	220
4.7	Critical voice record	221
4.8	Intrusive thoughts diary	222
4.9	OCD ritual diary	223
4.10	PTSD diary	224

5 Cognitive restructuring

5.1	Unhelpful thinking styles	225
5.2	Thought-disputing model	226
5.3	Decatastrophising model	227
5.4	Cost/benefit analysis	228
5.5	Worry tree	229
5.6	Theory A/B model	230
5.7	Health anxiety change model	231
5.8	Core belief challenging	232

5.9	Evidence table for core beliefs	*233*
5.10	Cycle of beliefs, rules and behaviours	*234*
5.11	Rules into values	*235*

6 Experiments

6.1	Behavioural experiment	*236*
6.2	Resilience-developing model	*237*
6.3	Worry time	*238*
6.4	Stimulus discrimination	*239*
6.5	Imagery-based exposure	*240*
6.6	Downward arrow model	*241*
6.7	Core belief experiment	*242*
6.8	Graded exposure for phobias	*243*
6.9	OCD graded exposure	*244*
6.10	Coping cards	*245*
6.11	Cognitive cue cards	*246*

7 Interpersonal strategies

7.1	Acknowledging needs	*247*
7.2	Thought record for assertiveness	*248*
7.3	Assertiveness technique log	*249*
7.4	Temperature reading	*250*
7.5	Circle of contact	*251*
7.6	Responsibility pie	*252*
7.7	Cycle of abuse	*253*

8 Relapse prevention

8.1	Improvement and impact reflection	*254*
8.2	New coping devices reflection	*255*
8.3	Progress not perfection charts	*256*
8.4	Early warning signs	*257*
8.5	Action plan	*258*
8.6	Future plans	*259*

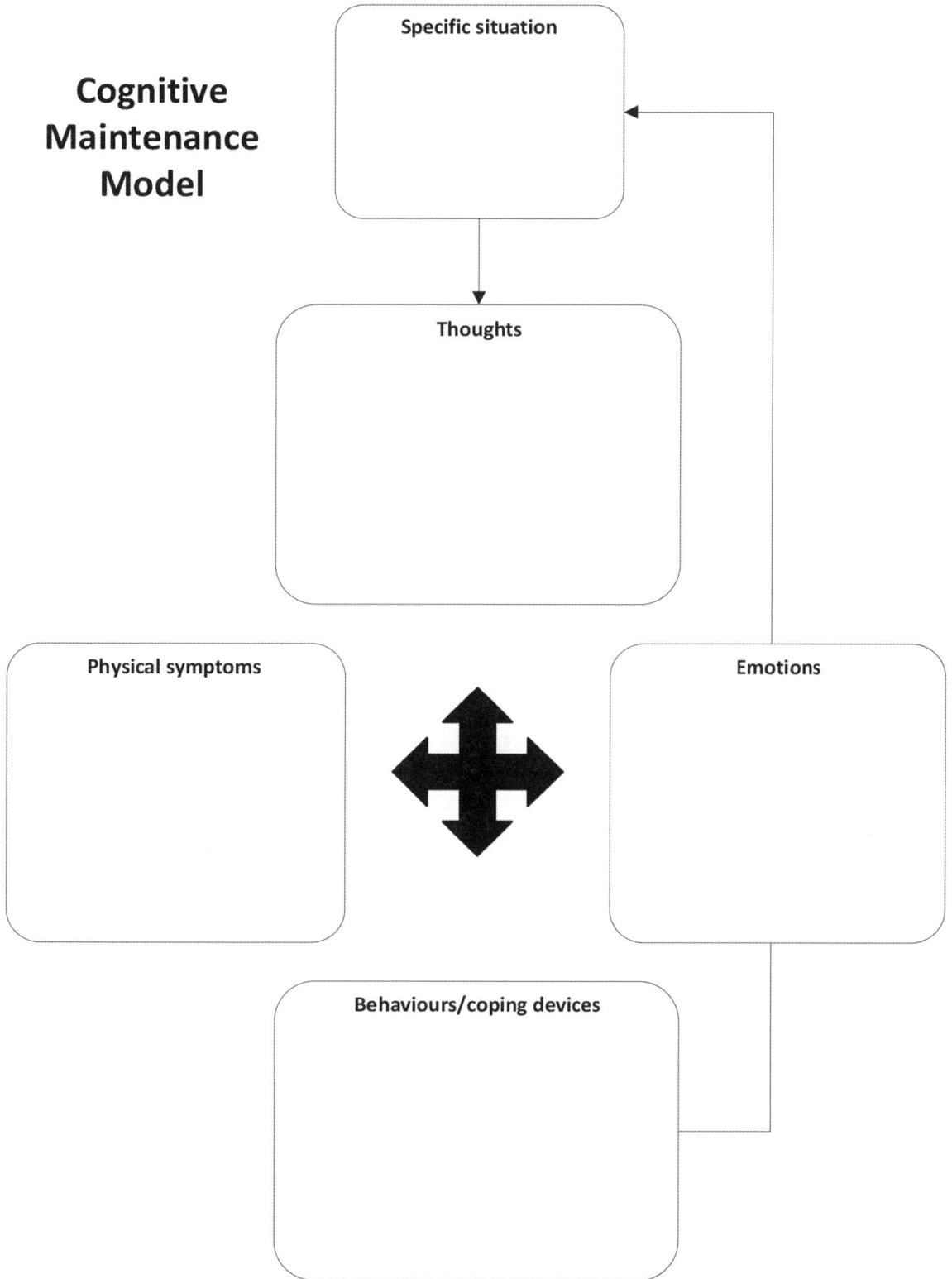

Cognitive Model of Panic

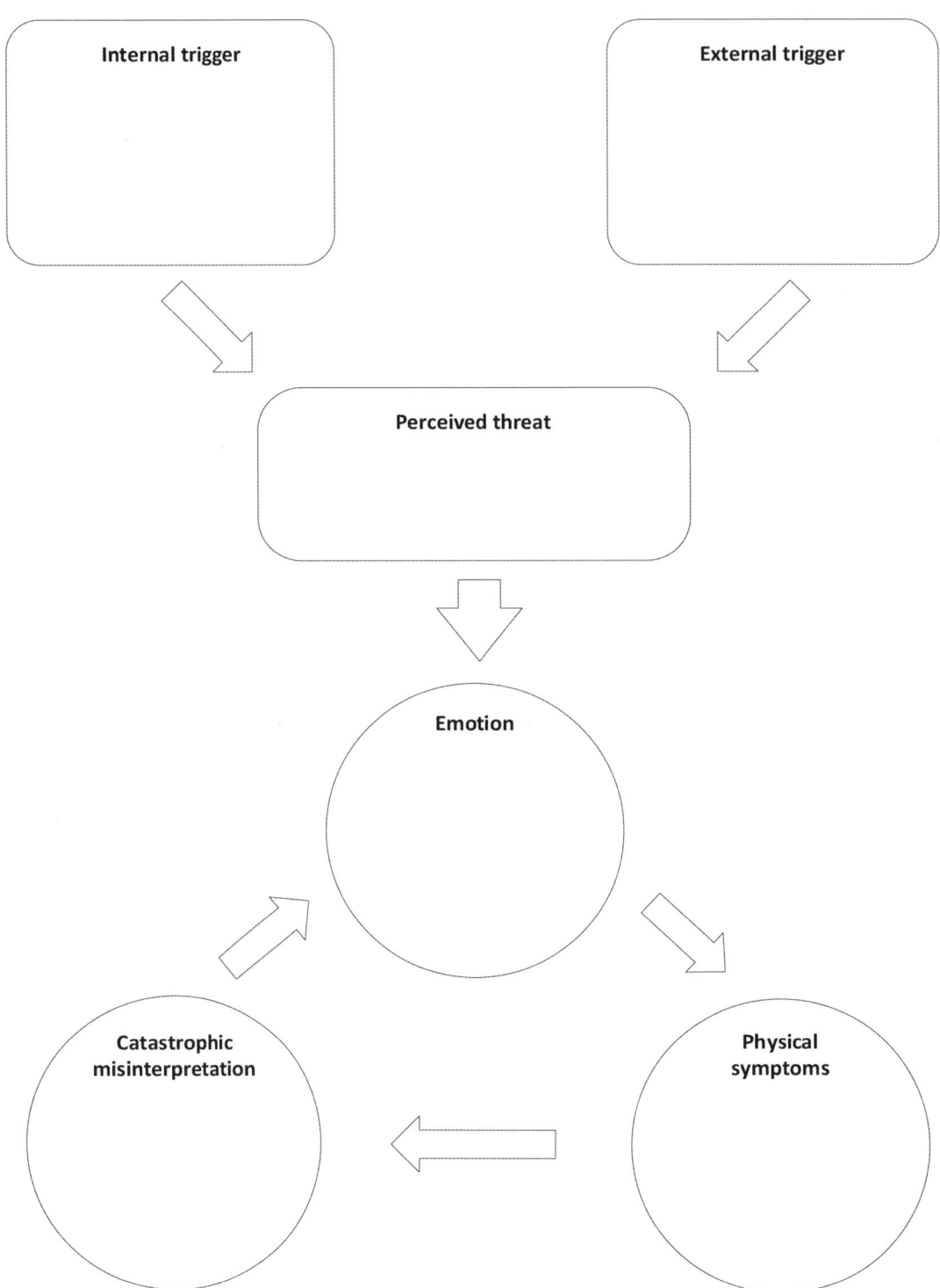

Cognitive Model of Perfectionism

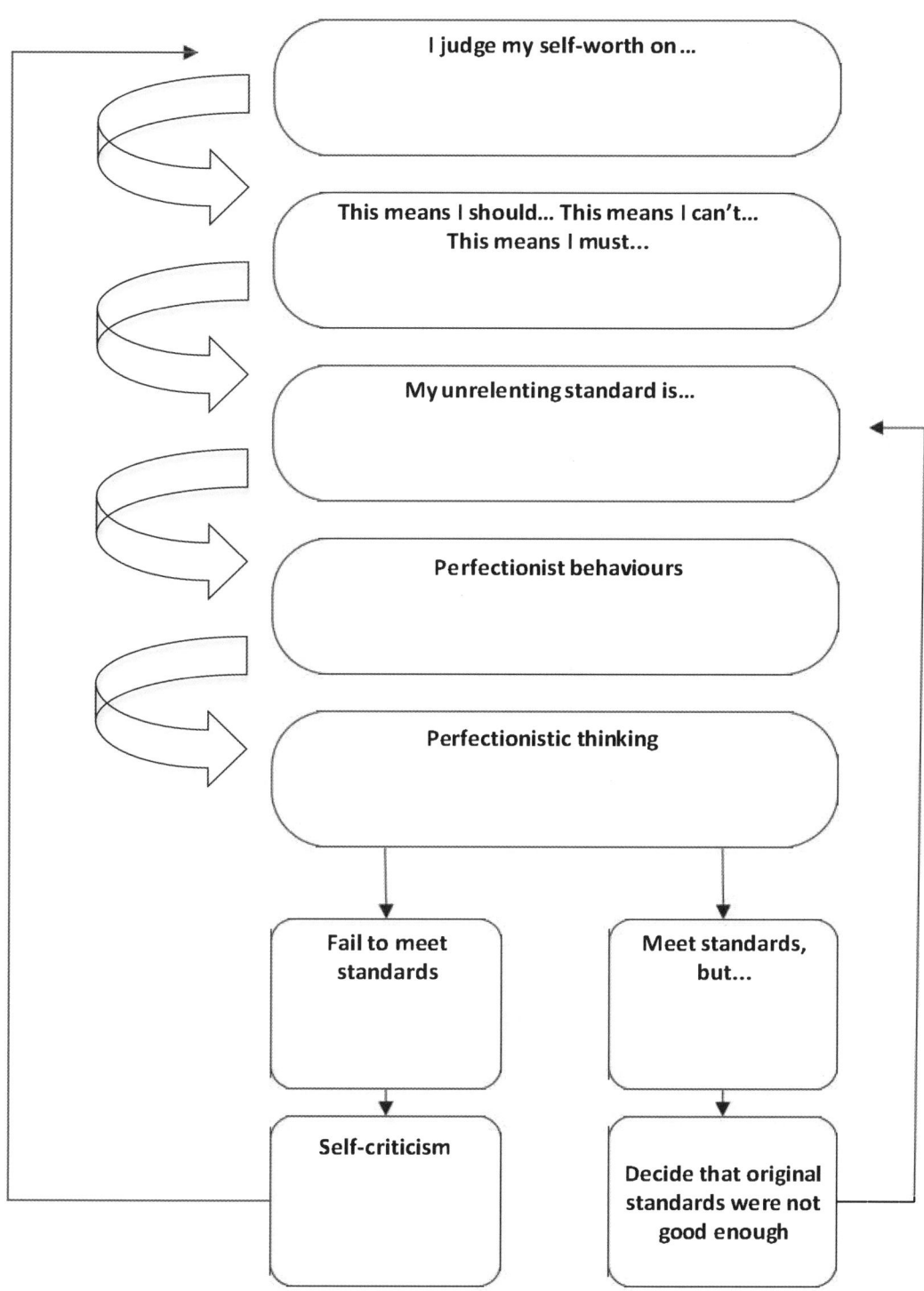

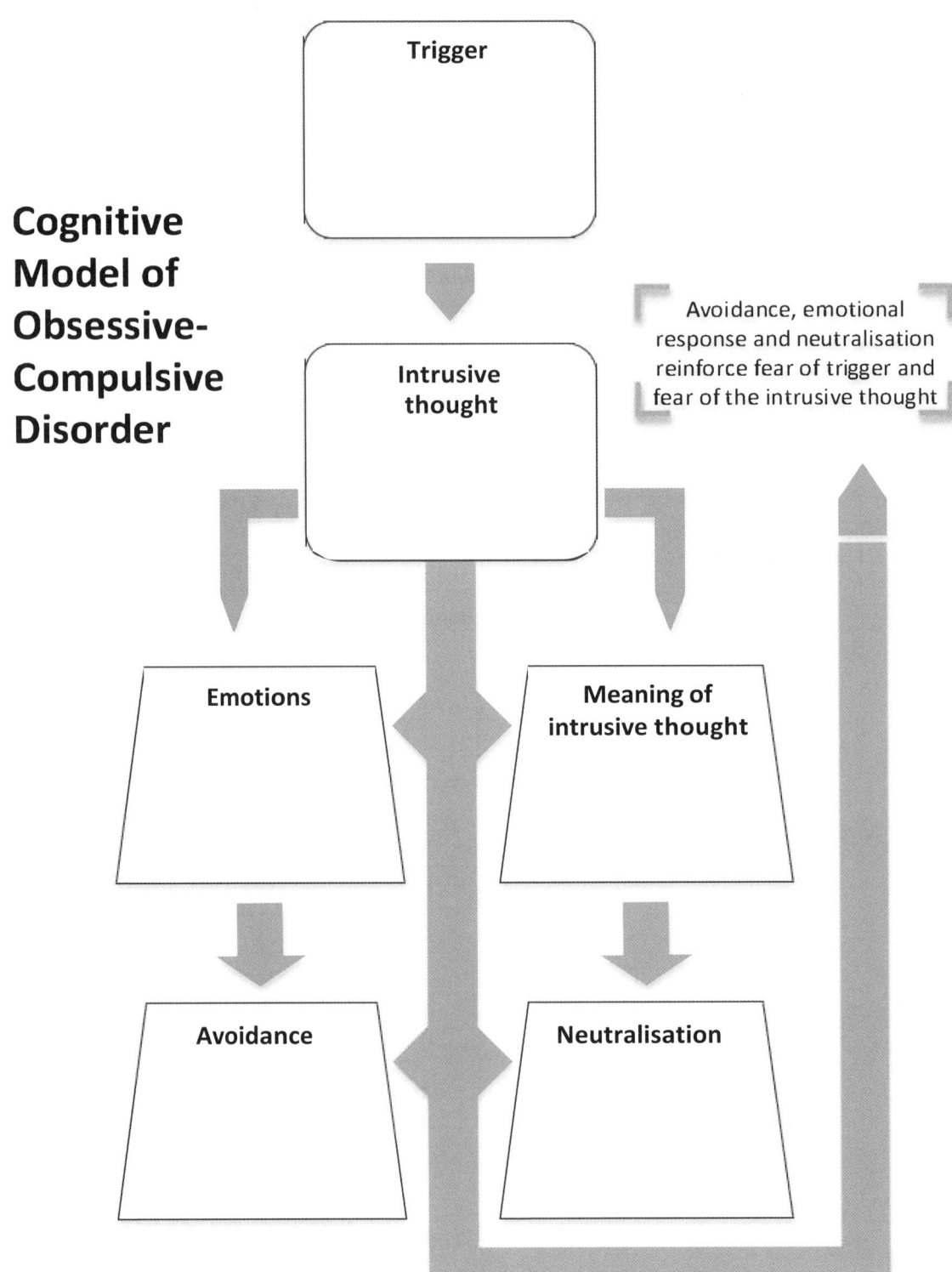

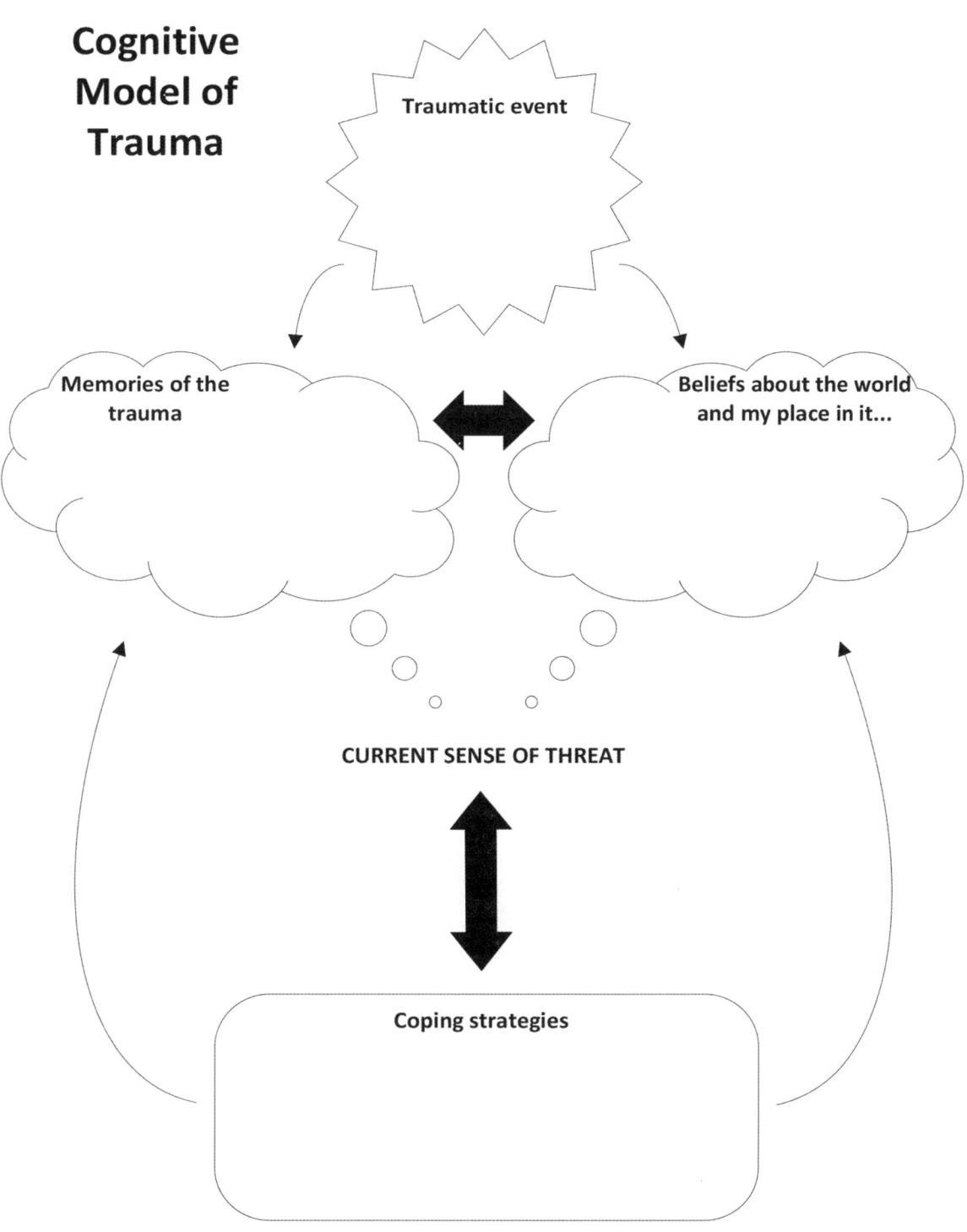

Vicious Flowers for Health Anxiety

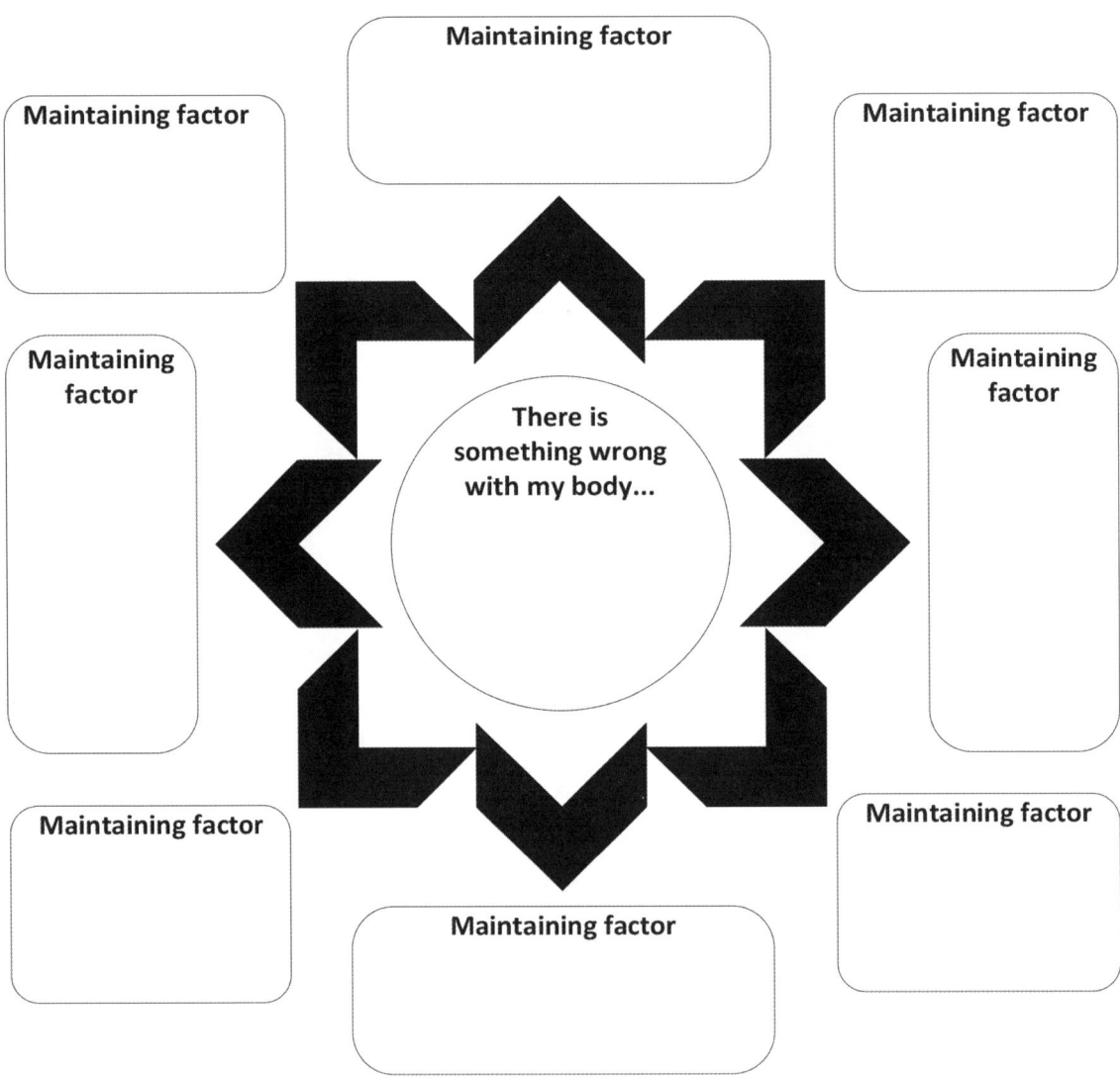

TRAP worksheet

Trigger — Event

Response — Thoughts/feelings

Avoidance **P**attern — Specific examples of behaviour that reduces the intensity of thoughts and feelings

Short-term consequences

Long-term consequences

TRAC worksheet

Trigger	**R**esponse	**A**lternative **C**oping
Event	Thoughts/feelings	Specific examples of behaviour that reduces the intensity of thoughts and feelings

Short-term consequences

Long-term consequences

Chapter 1. Formulations – Blank worksheets 193

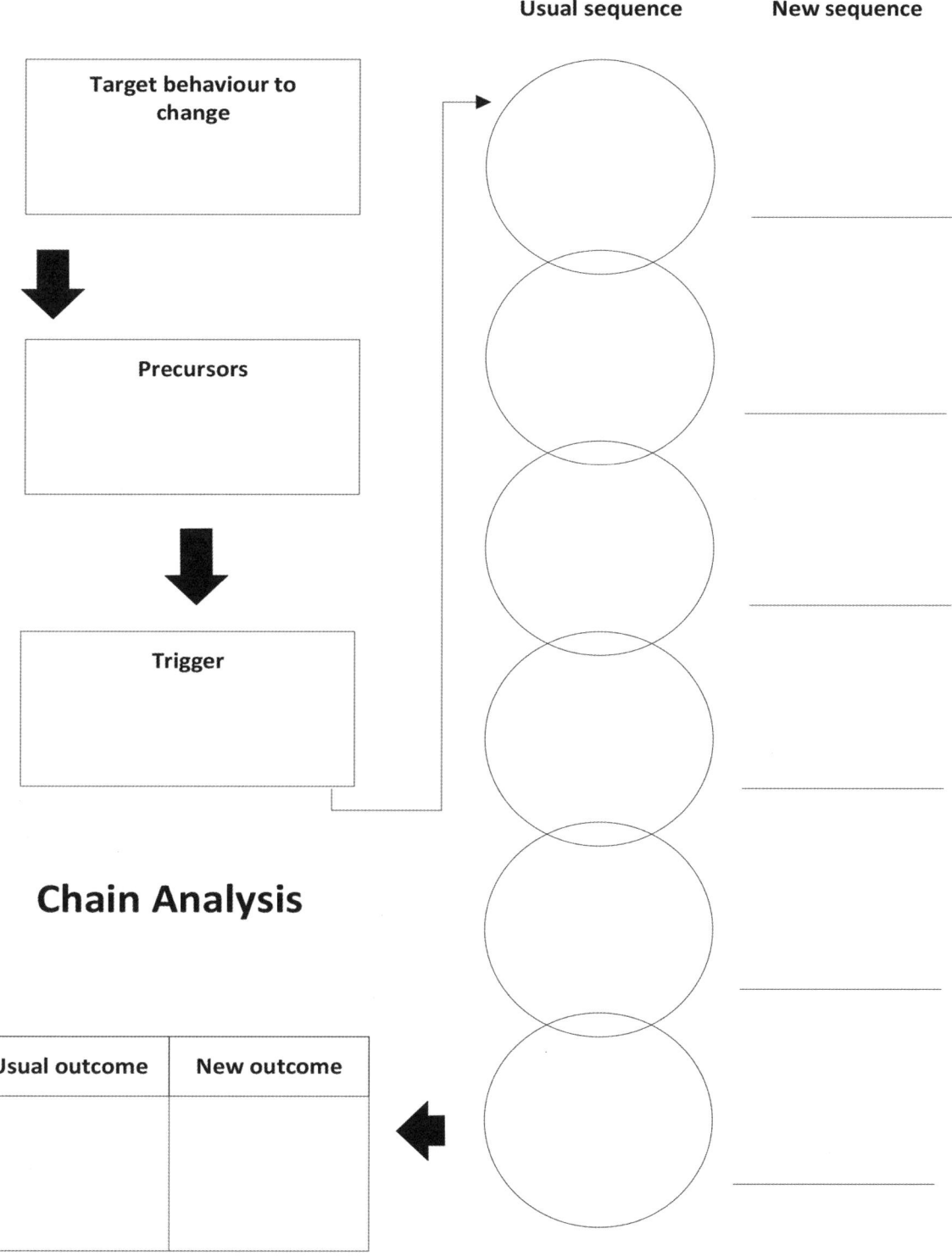

Chain Analysis

Chapter 1. Formulations – Blank worksheets

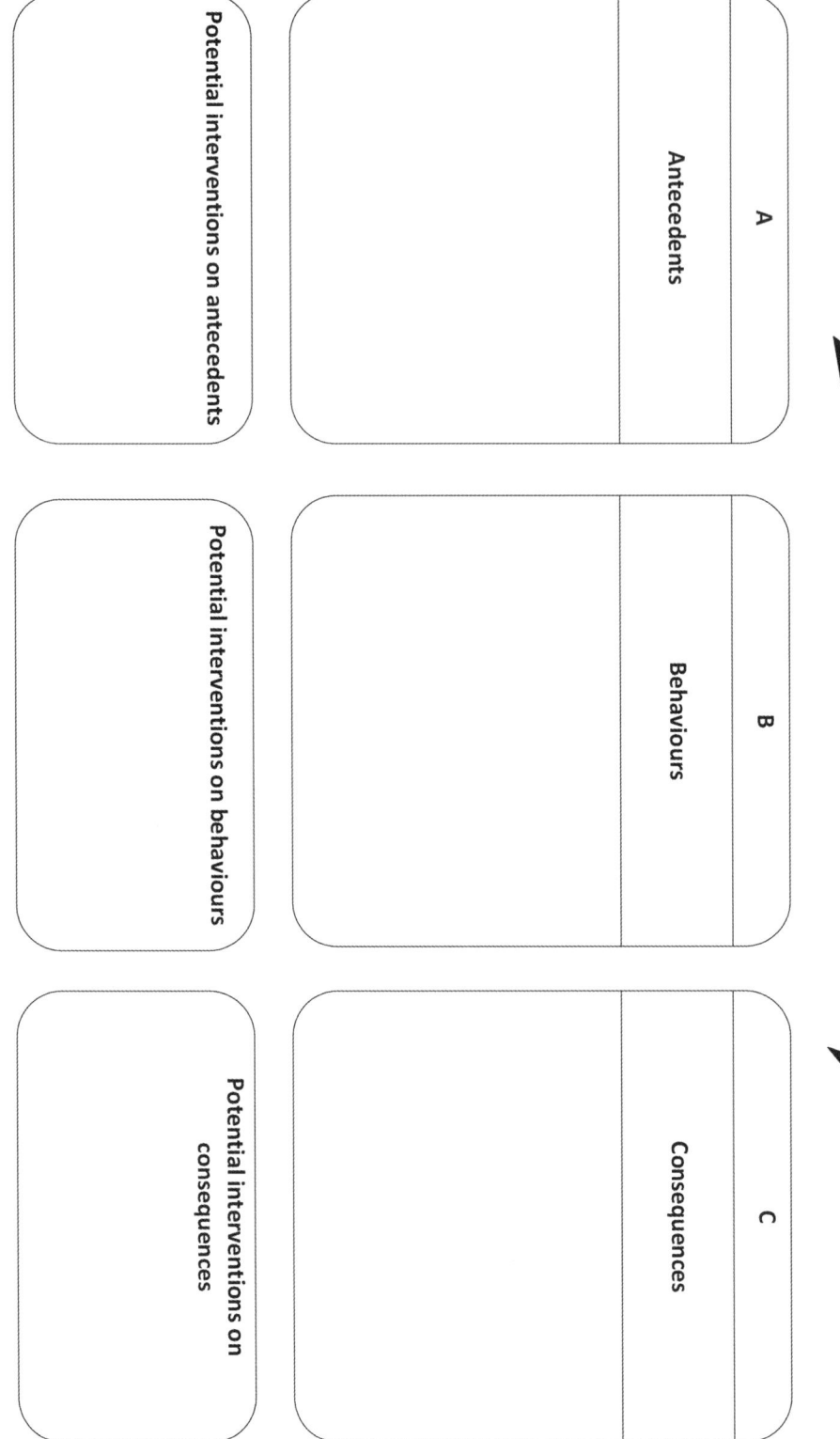

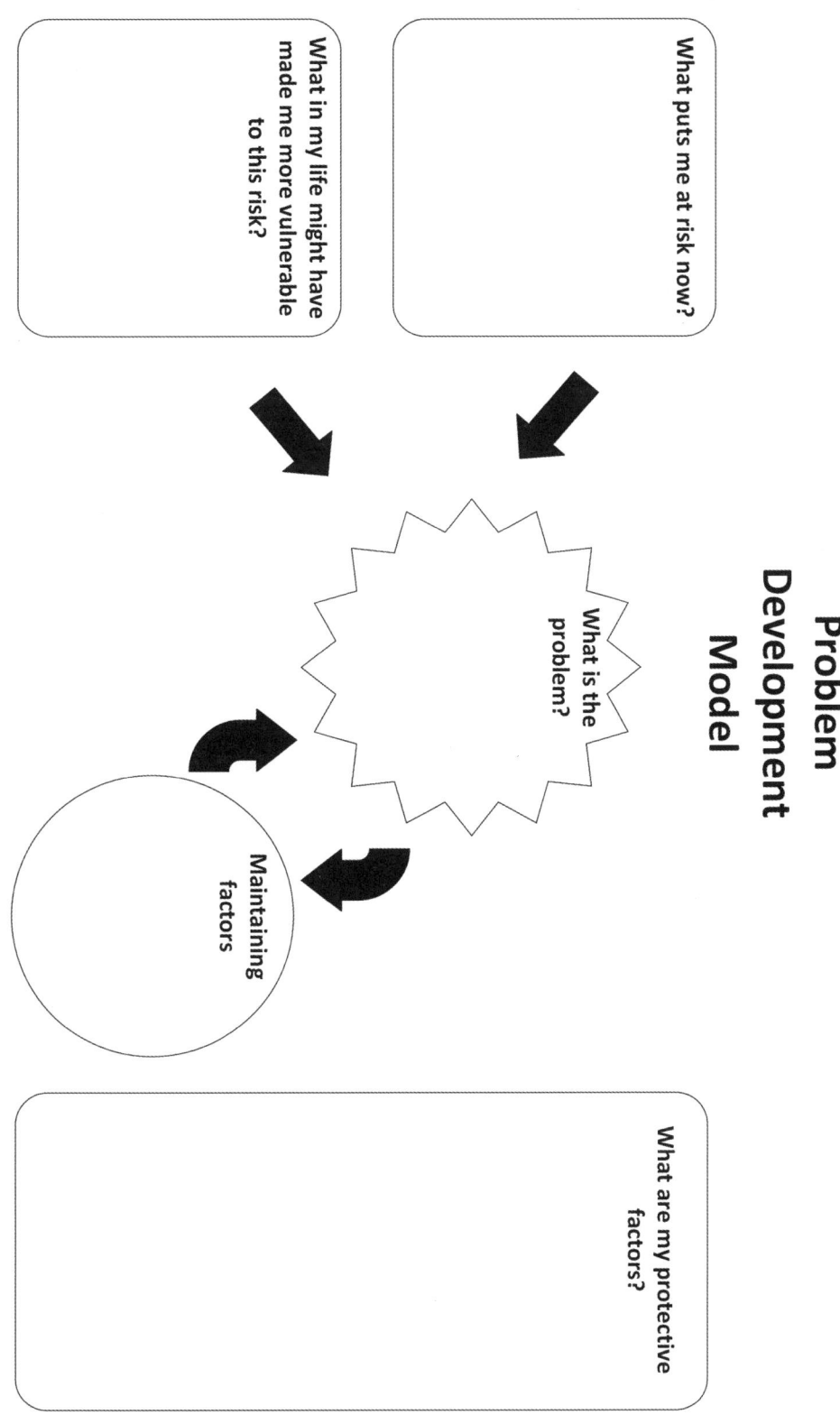

Coping Strategies Model

	Current problem

Unhealthy coping strategies	Consequences of unhealthy coping strategies

Potential healthy coping strategies	Expected outcomes of healthy coping strategies

Chapter 1. Formulations – Blank worksheets

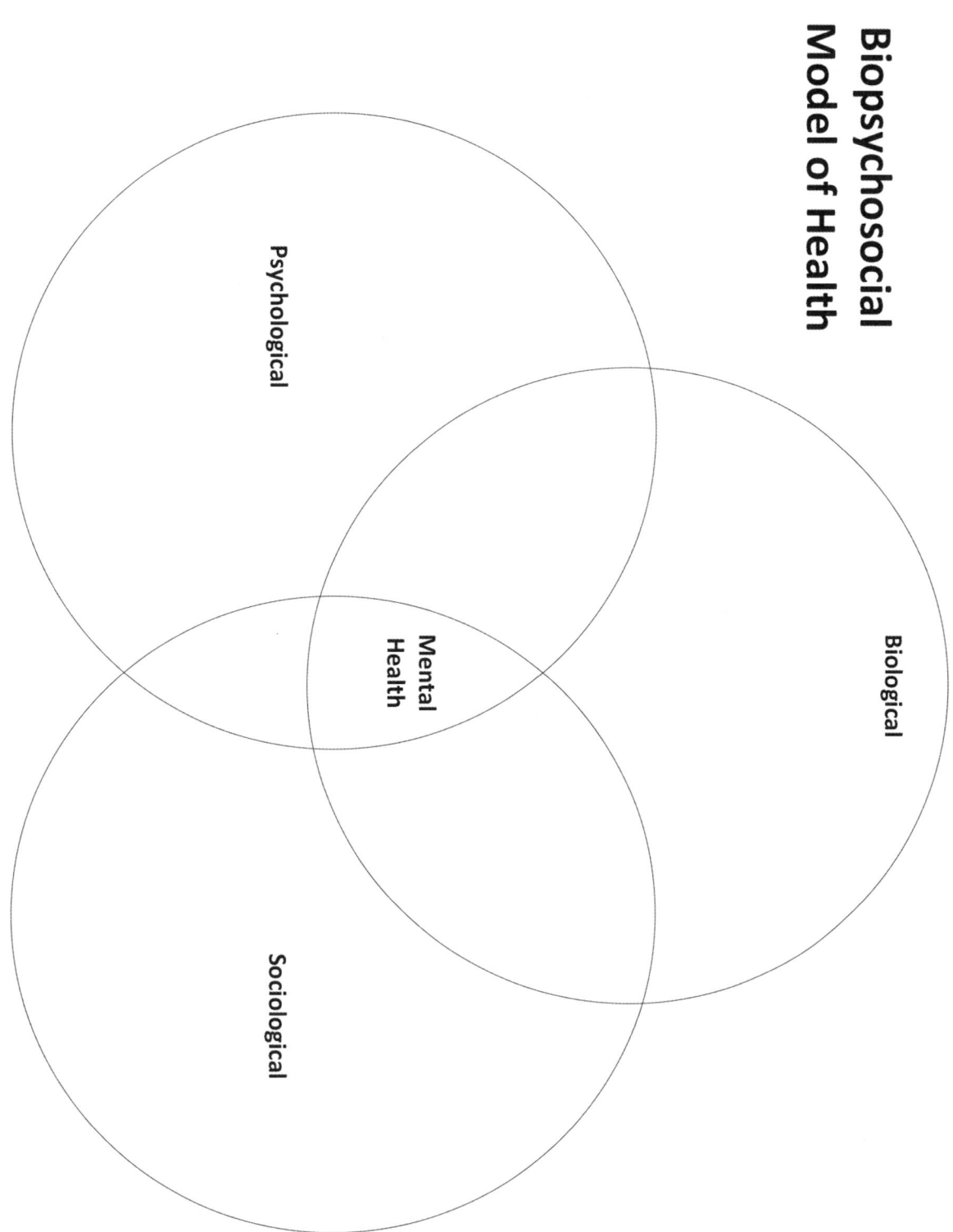

SMART Goals

Specific

Measurable

Achievable

Relevant

Time-limited

Nine Pillars

Contribution	Hobbies	Exercise
Family	Alone time	Personal growth
Work	Relationship	Friends

Sleep Hygiene Checkist

Sleep hygiene tips	No	Somewhat	Yes
Regular sleeping timetable			
Using the bed only for sleep			
Avoiding stimulating activities before sleep			
Avoiding caffeine and nicotine before sleep			
Avoiding alcohol before sleep			
No napping during the day			
Having an evening ritual			
Avoiding hot baths before sleep			
No clock watching			
Using a sleep diary/app			
Exercising during the day			
Avoiding exercise 4 hours before sleep			
Eating a balanced, nutritious diet			
Making sure the bedroom is dark when sleeping			
Making sure to do activities during the day even if tired			

Initial sleeping goals

Reality vs Expectations

Improve my reality	Change my expectations

Stress Quadrant

Important and urgent	**Important and not urgent**
Not important and urgent	**Not important and not urgent**

Phobia Ladder

Fear rating	Activity hierarchy	0–100
Most feared – 75–100		
Medium feared – 50–75		
Least feared – 20–50		

Behavioural Diary

	Monday	Tuesday	Wednesday	Thursday	Friday	Saturday	Sunday
Morning What: Where: Who:							
Morning What: Where: Who:							
Afternoon What: Where: Who:							
Afternoon What: Where: Who:							
Evening What: Where: Who:							
Evening What: Where: Who:							

Identifying Activities

Routine

Pleasurable

Necessary

⬇

Easiest

Medium

Hardest

Alternative Solutions Model

Specific problem:			
Possible solution	**Strengths**	**Weaknesses**	**Yes/no**

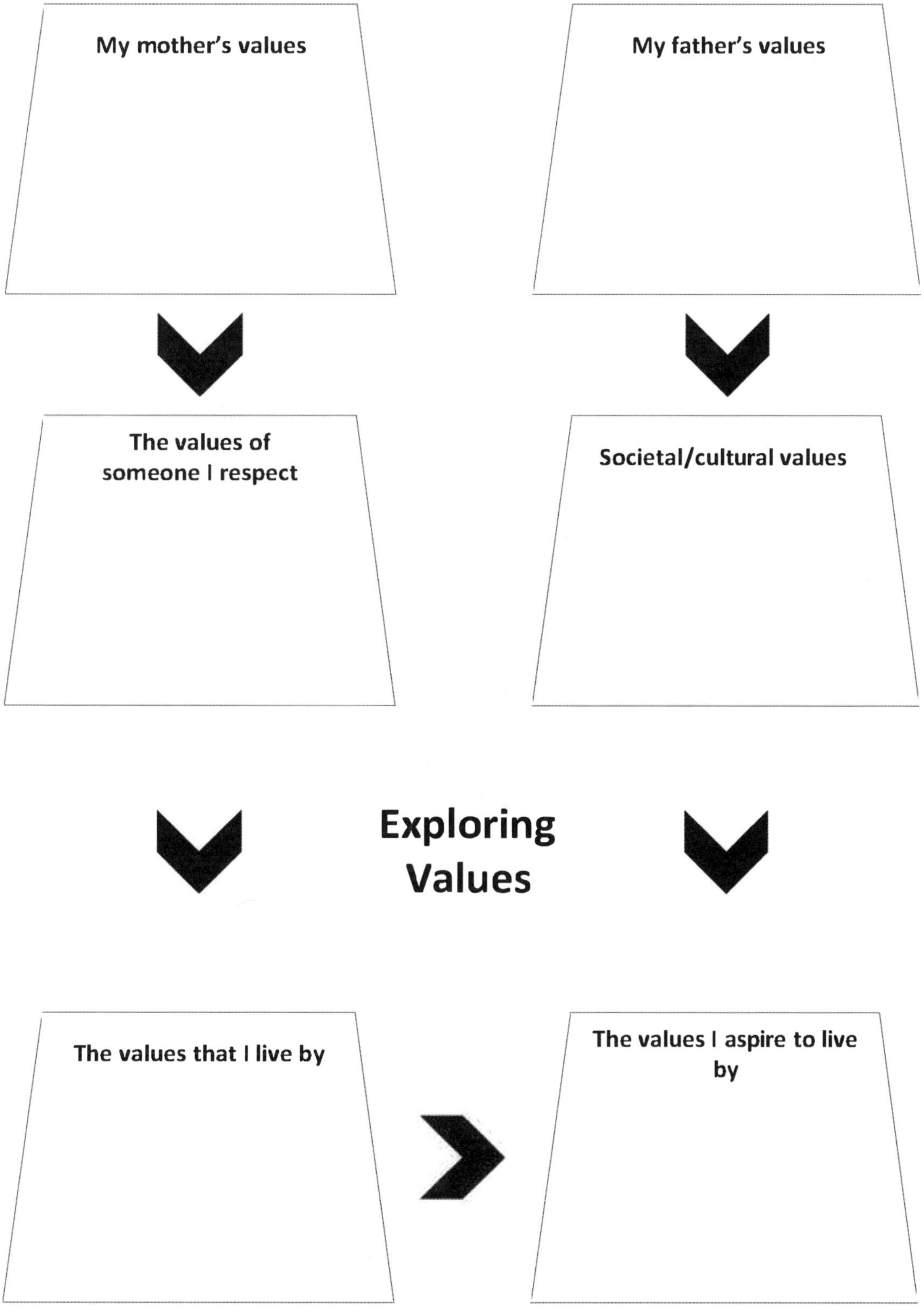

Chapter 2. Goals and behavioural planning – Blank worksheets 207

My mother's values	My father's values
▼	▼
The values of someone I respect	Societal/cultural values

Exploring Values

The values that I live by	▶	The values I aspire to live by

208 Chapter 2. Goals and behavioural planning – Blank worksheets

Value Compass

Name of value:

Towards your value… →

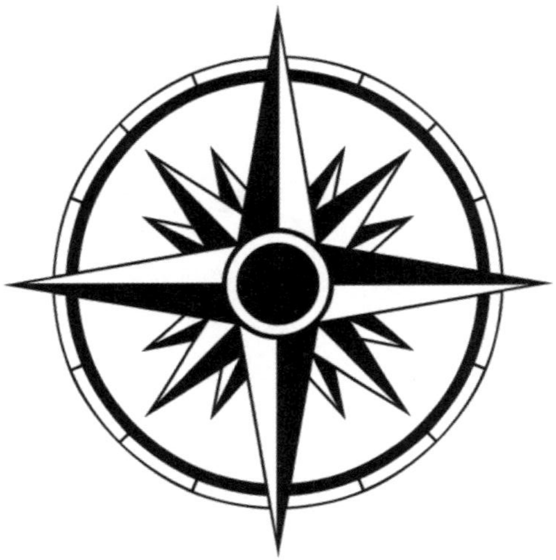

Away from your value… ←

Square Breathing Technique

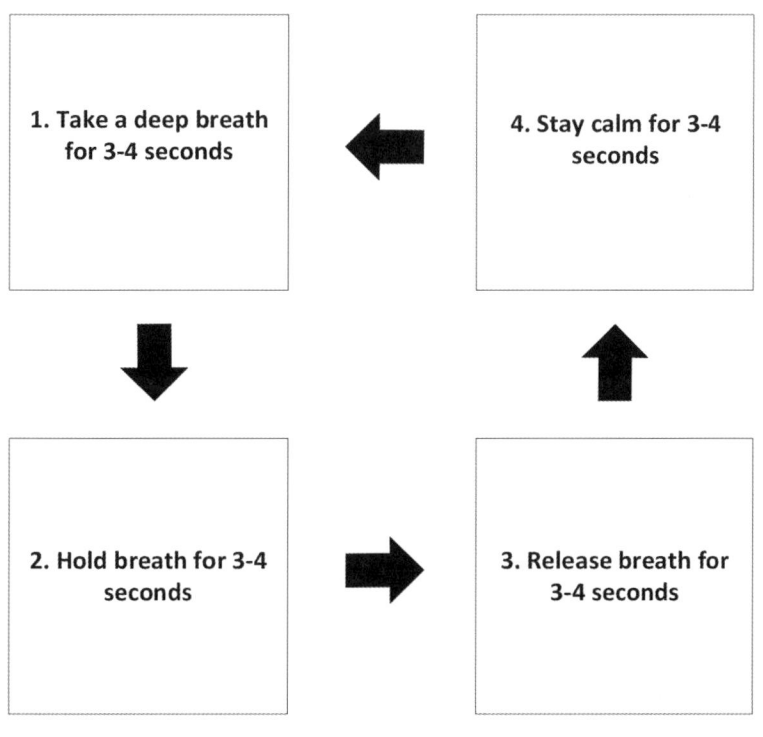

Reflections

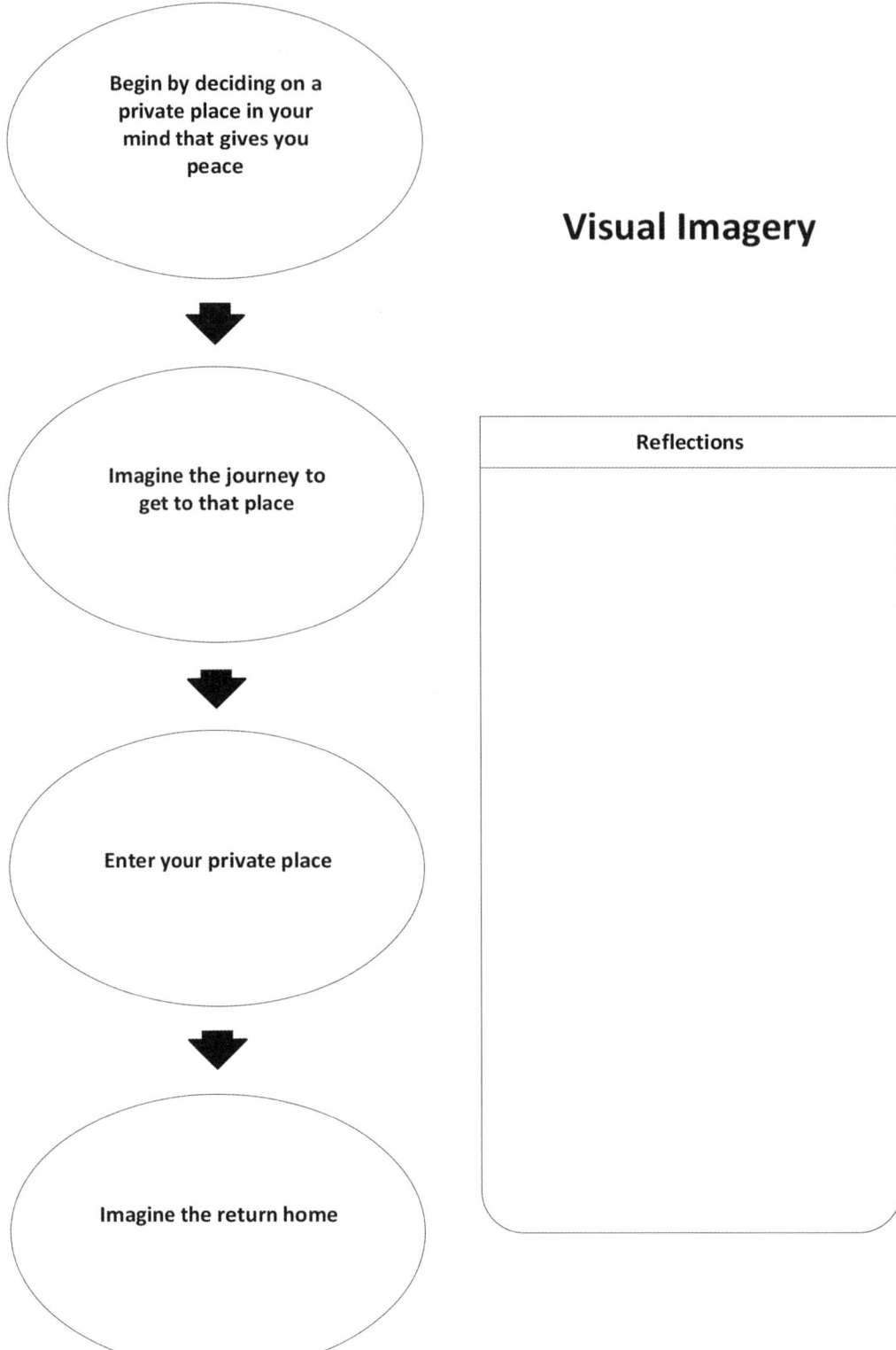

Progressive Muscle Relaxation

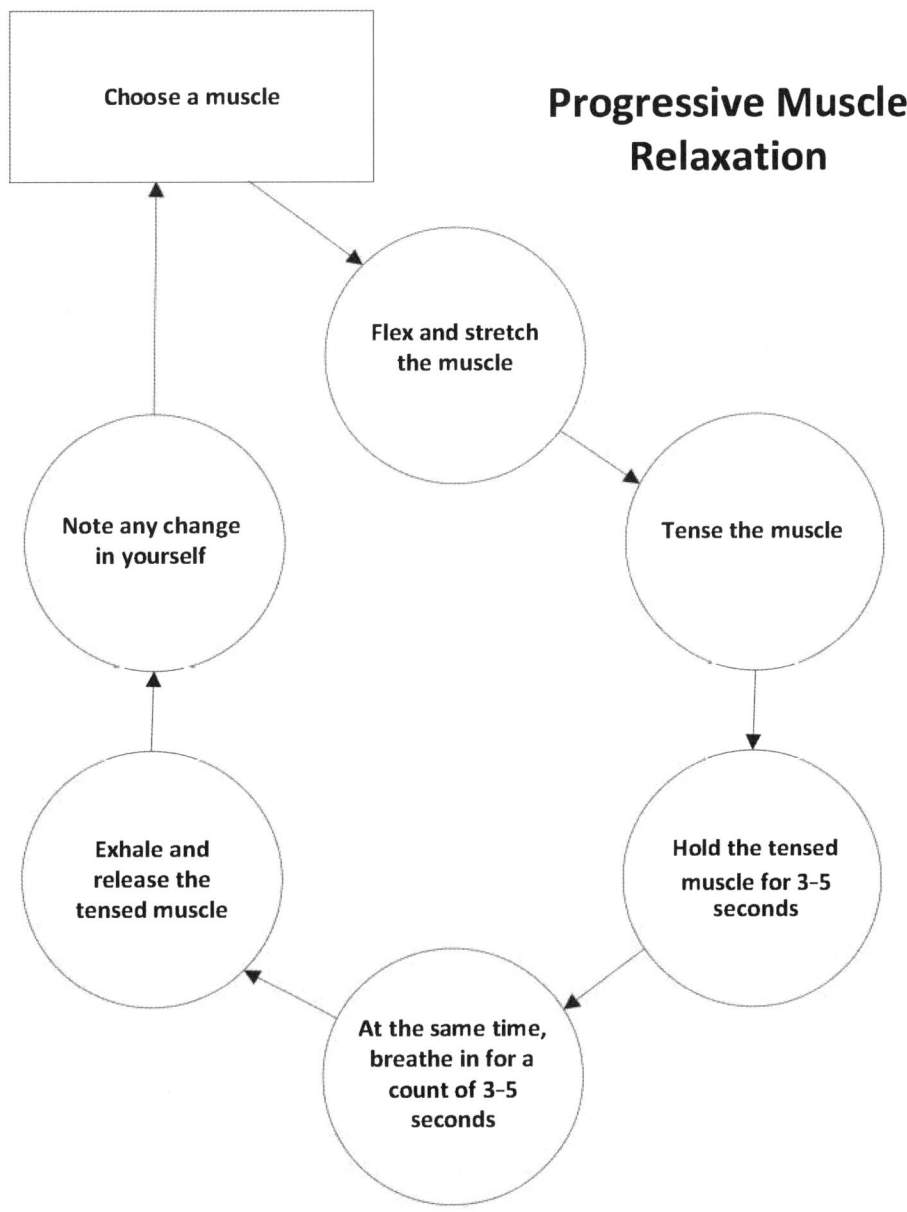

Reflections

212   Chapter 3. Relaxation – Blank worksheets

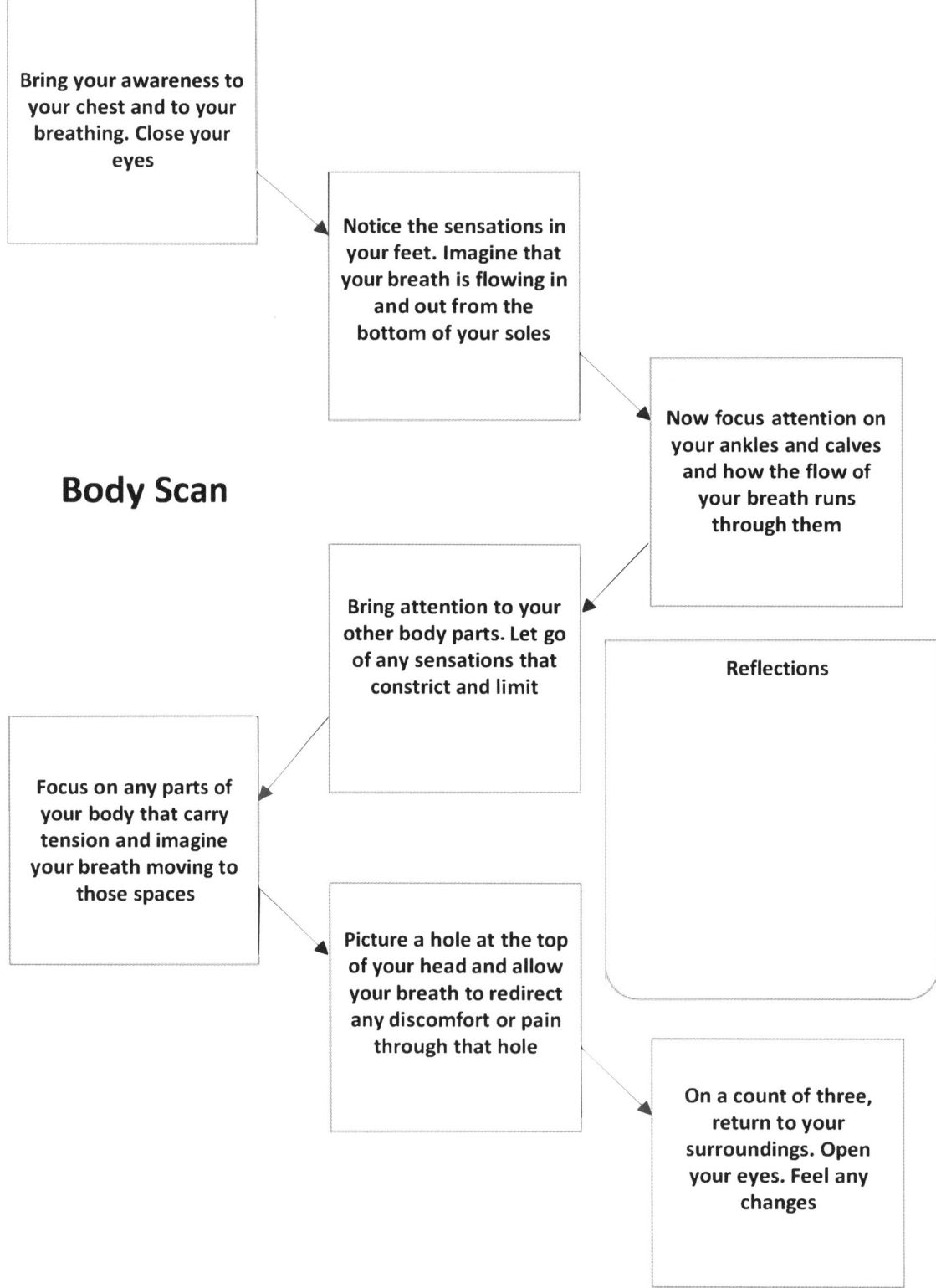

Mundane Task Focusing

Mundane tasks

Self-focused attention	%
Task-focused attention	%

Engage in chosen mundane task: if attention wanders, focus on all five senses

Self-focused attention	%
Task-focused attention	%

Grounding

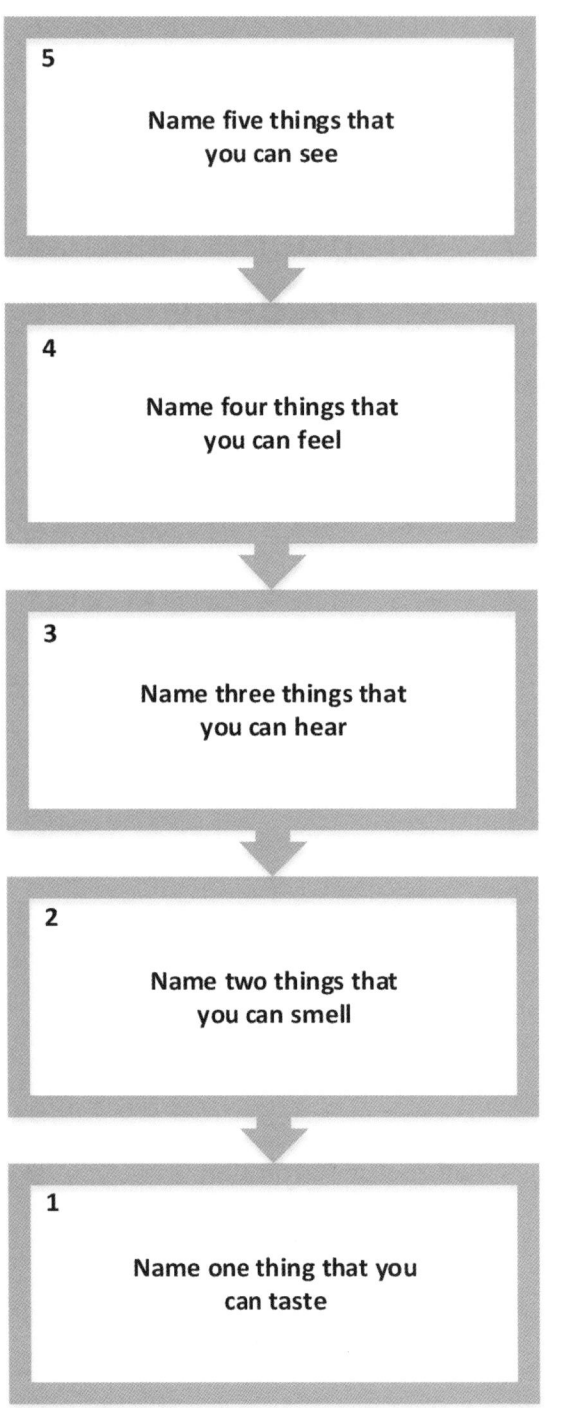

Reflections

Worry Diary

Situation	Thoughts	What do you fear might happen?	Emotions	Not important	Important and can be solved	Important but cannot be solved

Problematic Behaviour Diary

Trigger	Behaviour	Consequences of behaviour	Potential new behaviour	Potential new consequences of behaviour	Reflection

Relaxation Diary

Situation	Anxiety before %	Relaxation technique	Time spent using technique	Anxiety after %

Food Journal

	Breakfast	Lunch	Dinner	Snacks	Drinks
Monday					
Tuesday					
Wednesday					
Thursday					
Friday					
Saturday					
Sunday					

Panic Diary

Situation	Intensity %	Physical symptoms	Feared consequences	Behaviour	Actual consequences	Alternative explanation

Health Anxiety Thought Record

Date/time	Trigger	Emotion	Negative thought	How I responded	Rational response to negative thought

Critical Voice Record

Situation	Self-critical thought	Emotion	Belief in critical thought %	Self-compassionate alternative thought

Intrusive Thoughts Diary

Trigger/situation	Intrusive thought	Interpretation of intrusive thought	Behaviour to reduce intensity of intrusive thought

OCD Ritual Diary

Situation/time	Description of ritual	Discomfort felt %	Duration of ritual

PTSD Diary

Situation	Emotion	Physical reaction	Distorted thoughts/ images	Realistic assessment	New response

Unhelpful Thinking Styles

Situation	Thought	Emotions	My unhelpful thinking styles

Chapter 5. Cognitive restructuring – Blank worksheets

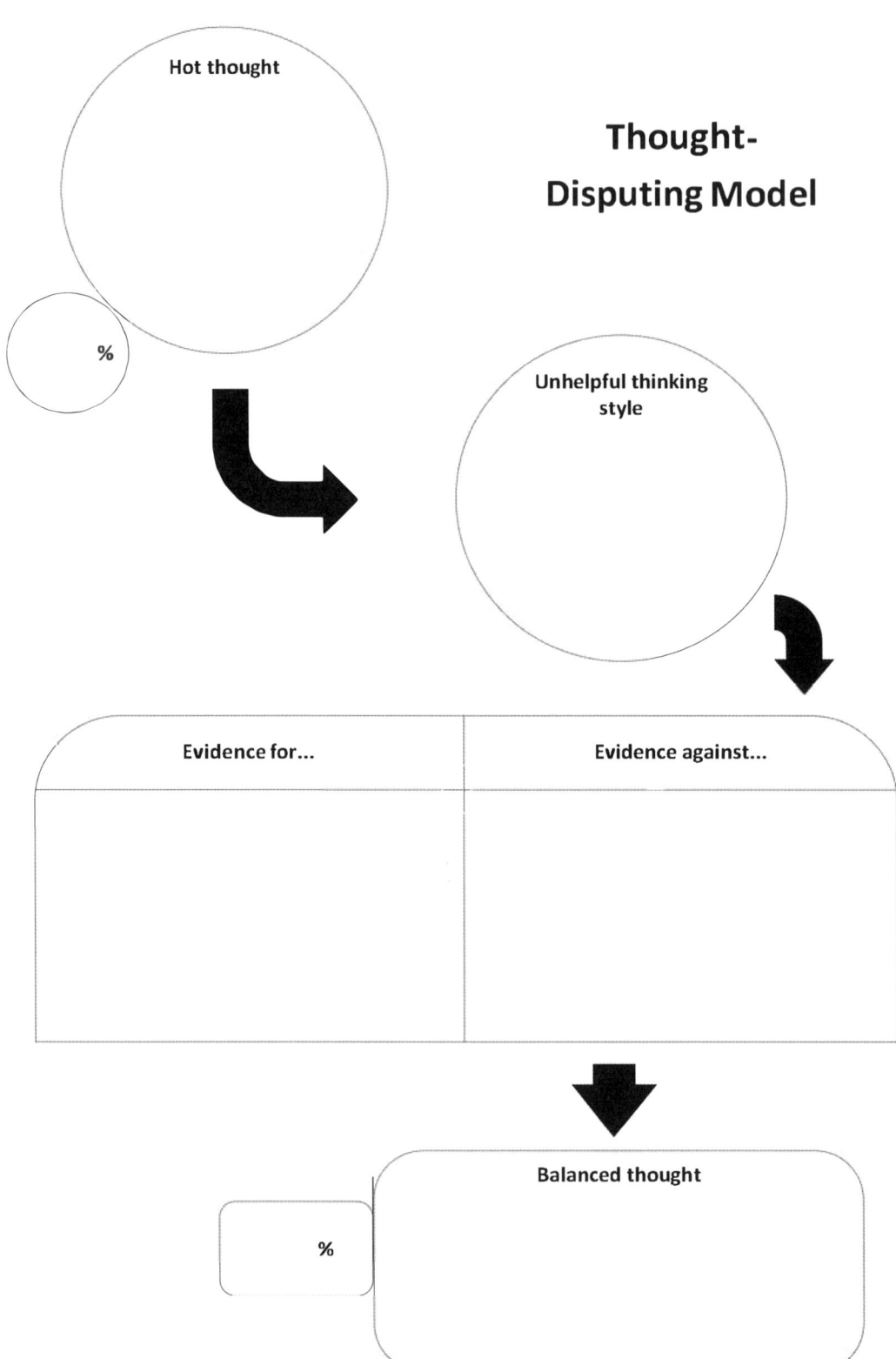

Chapter 5. Cognitive restructuring – Blank worksheets 227

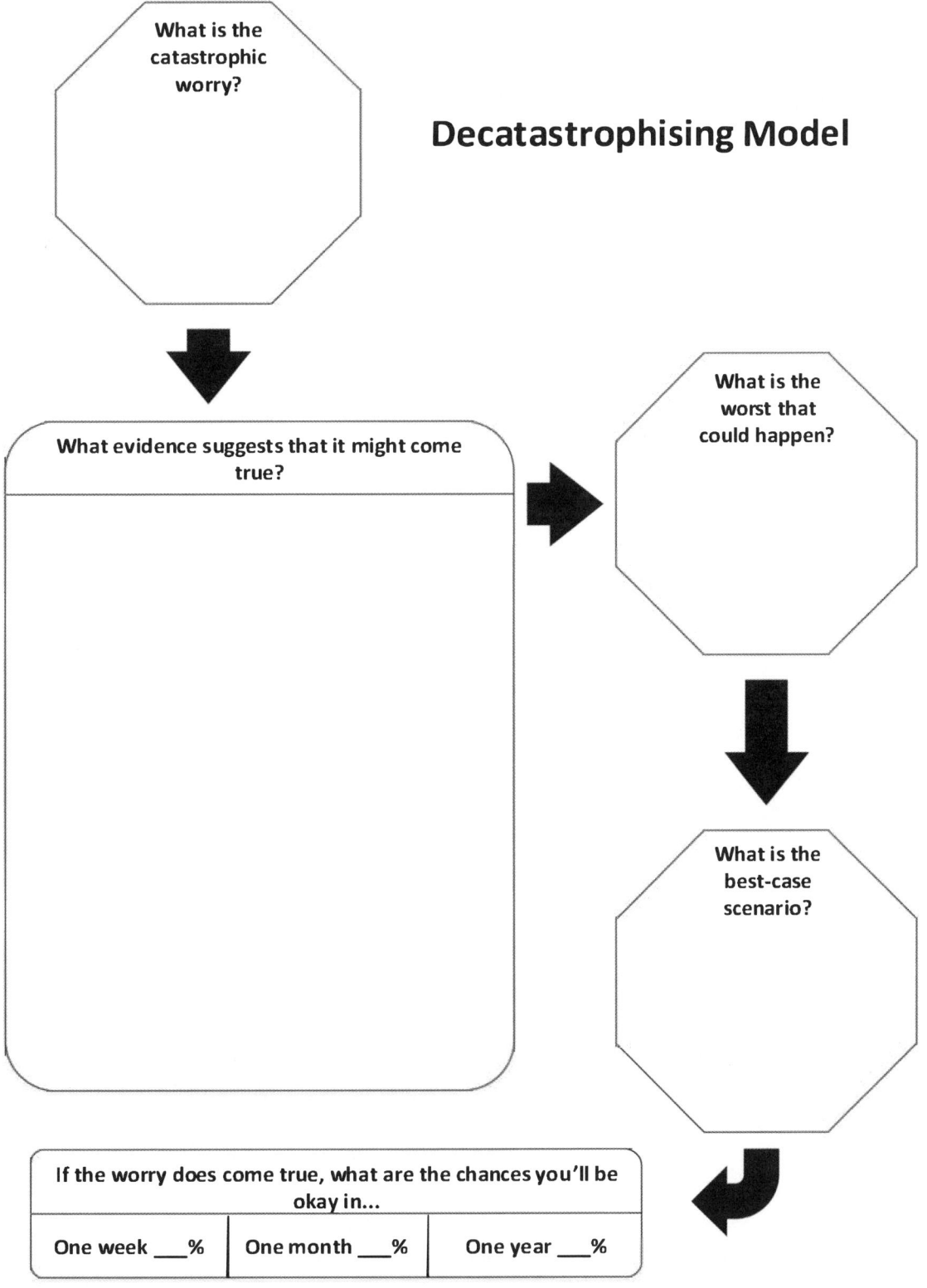

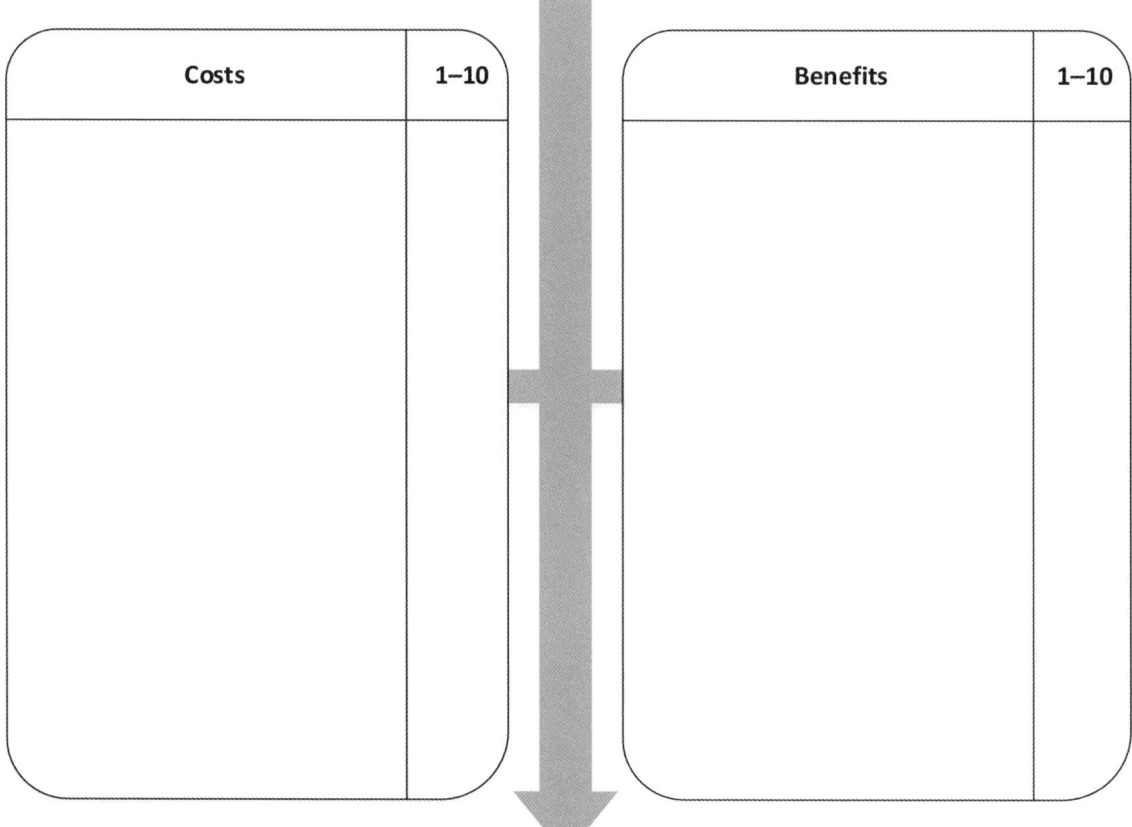

Worry Tree

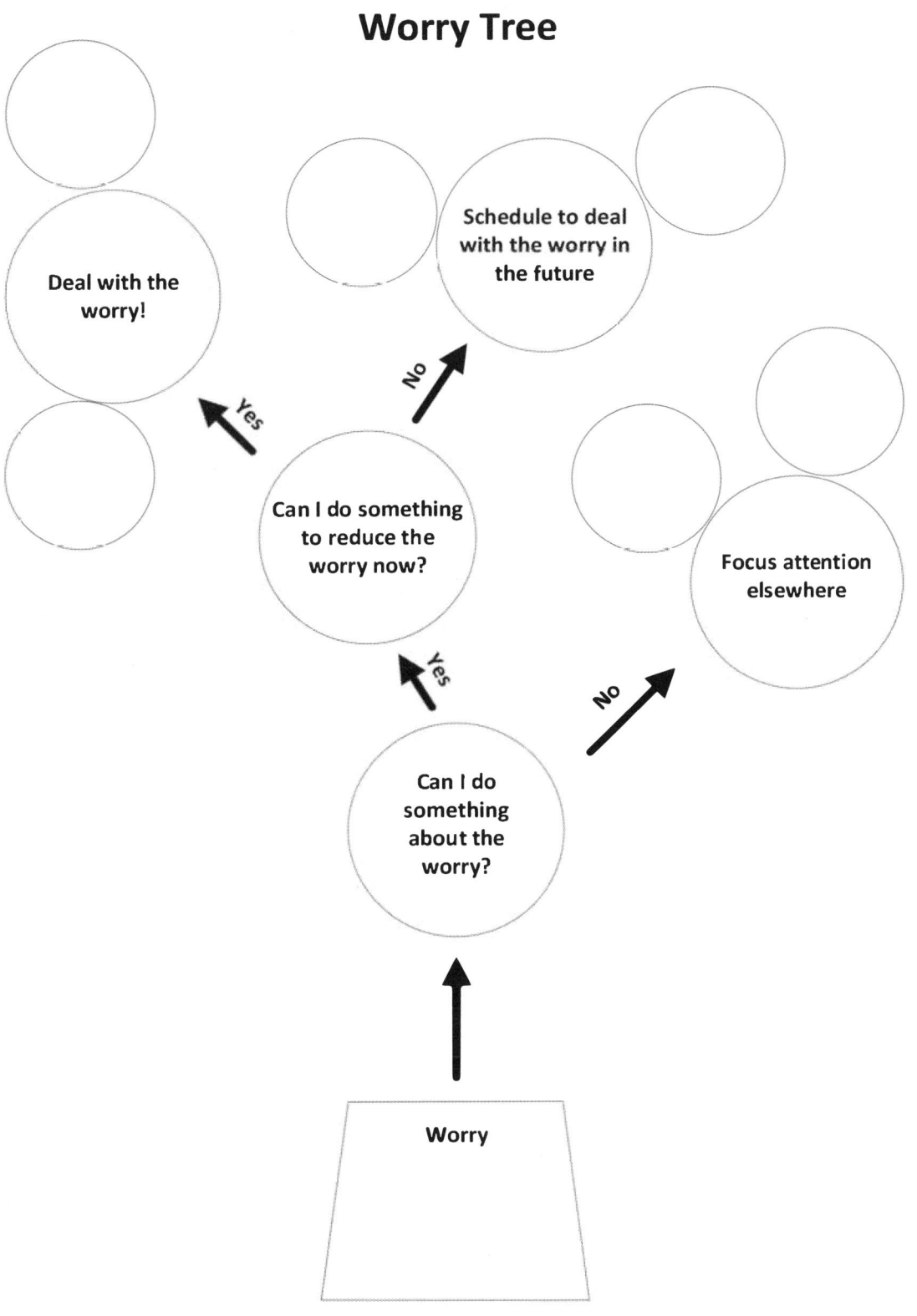

Theory A/B Model

Theory A	Theory B
The problem is...	**The problem is self-doubt, worry, rumination that...**
What is the hard evidence that this is true?	**What is the hard evidence that this is true?**
What do I need to do if theory A is true?	**What do I need to do if theory B is true?**

Chapter 5. Cognitive restructuring – Blank worksheets   231

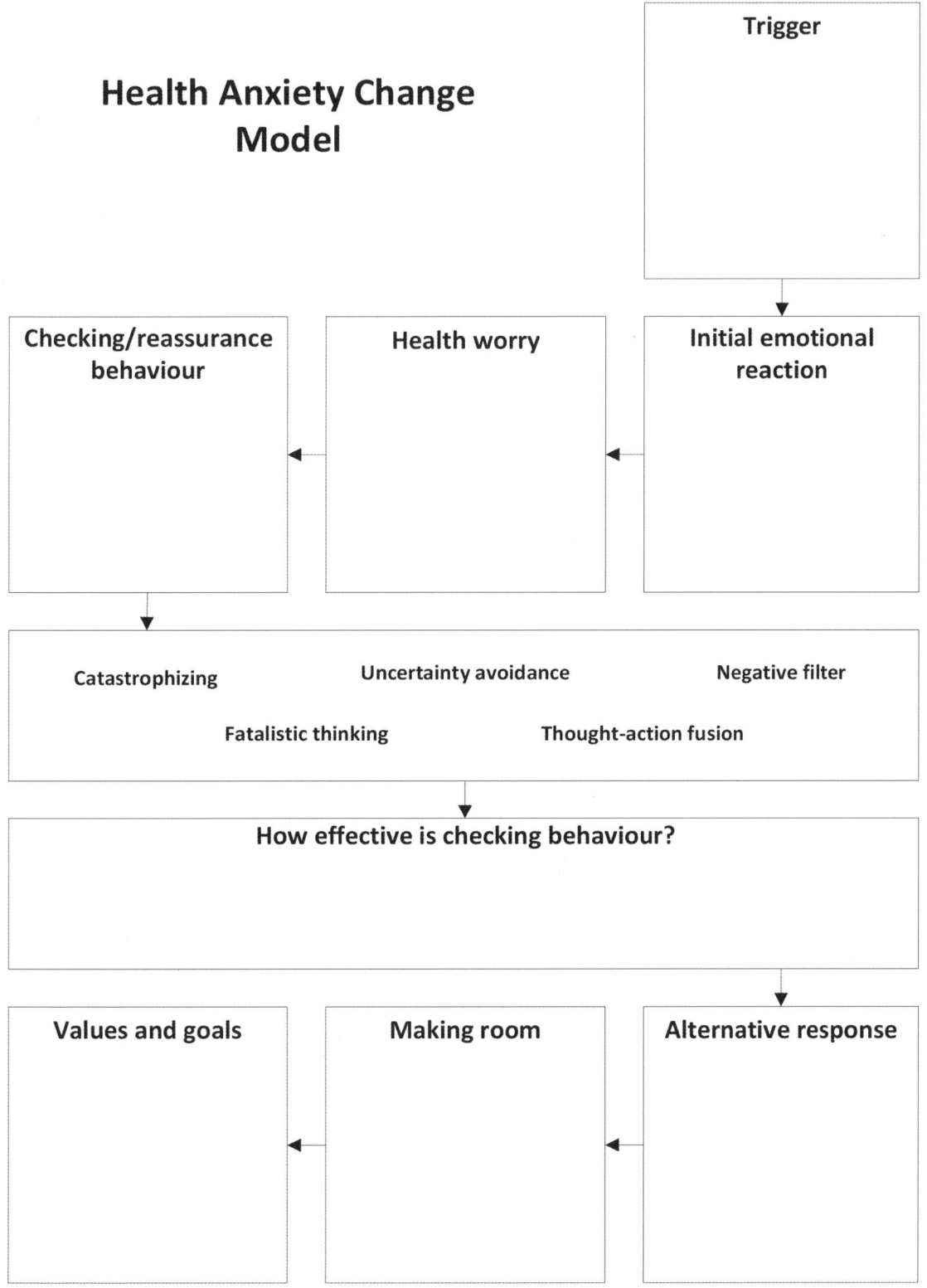

Core Belief Challenging

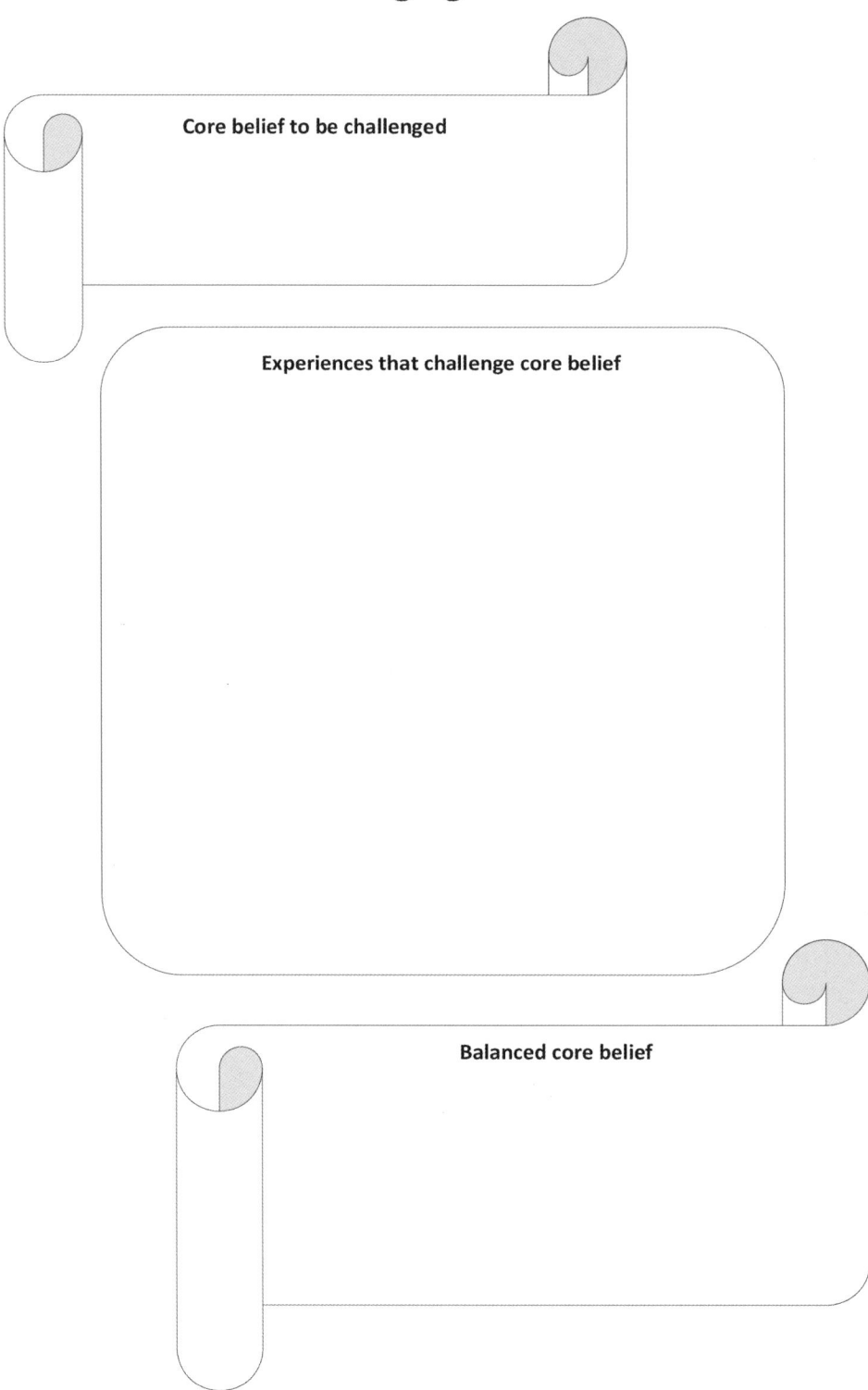

Evidence Table for Core Beliefs

Unhealthy core belief

Healthy core belief

Cycle of Beliefs, Rules and Behaviours

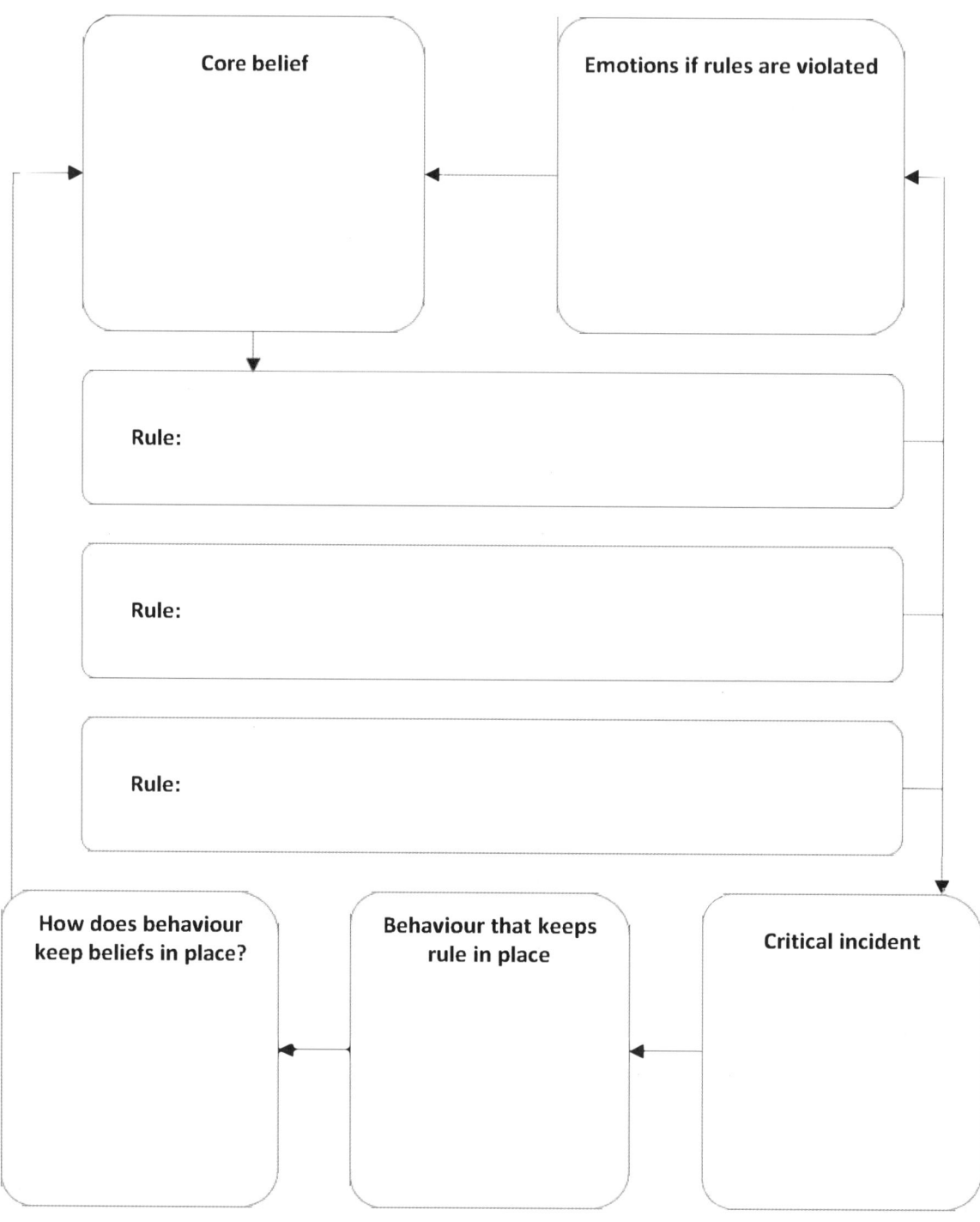

Rules into Values

Personal, self-limiting rule	Unhelpful outcome of applying rule	Personal value behind rule	Flexible way of applying rule

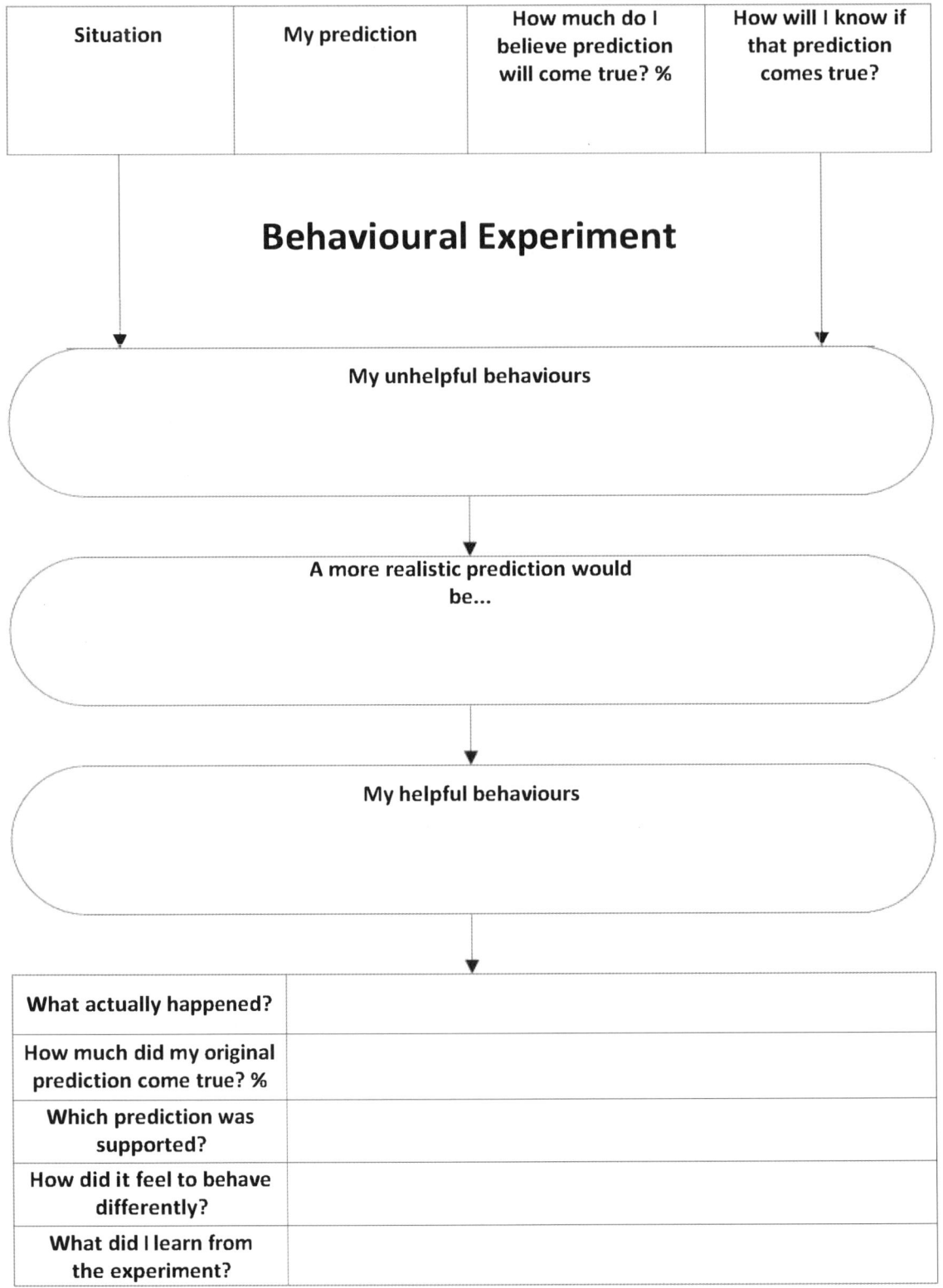

Resilience-Developing Model

Where would you like to enhance your resilience?

Strategies to put into action	How to apply strategies for this specific challenge

What would resilience look like?	
How would resilience feel?	

Results of applying strategies

Worry Time

My daily worry time is _____   **Length of time worrying** _____

| **Post-worry time pleasurable activity** | **Weekly worry review** |

Chapter 6. Experiments – Blank worksheets 239

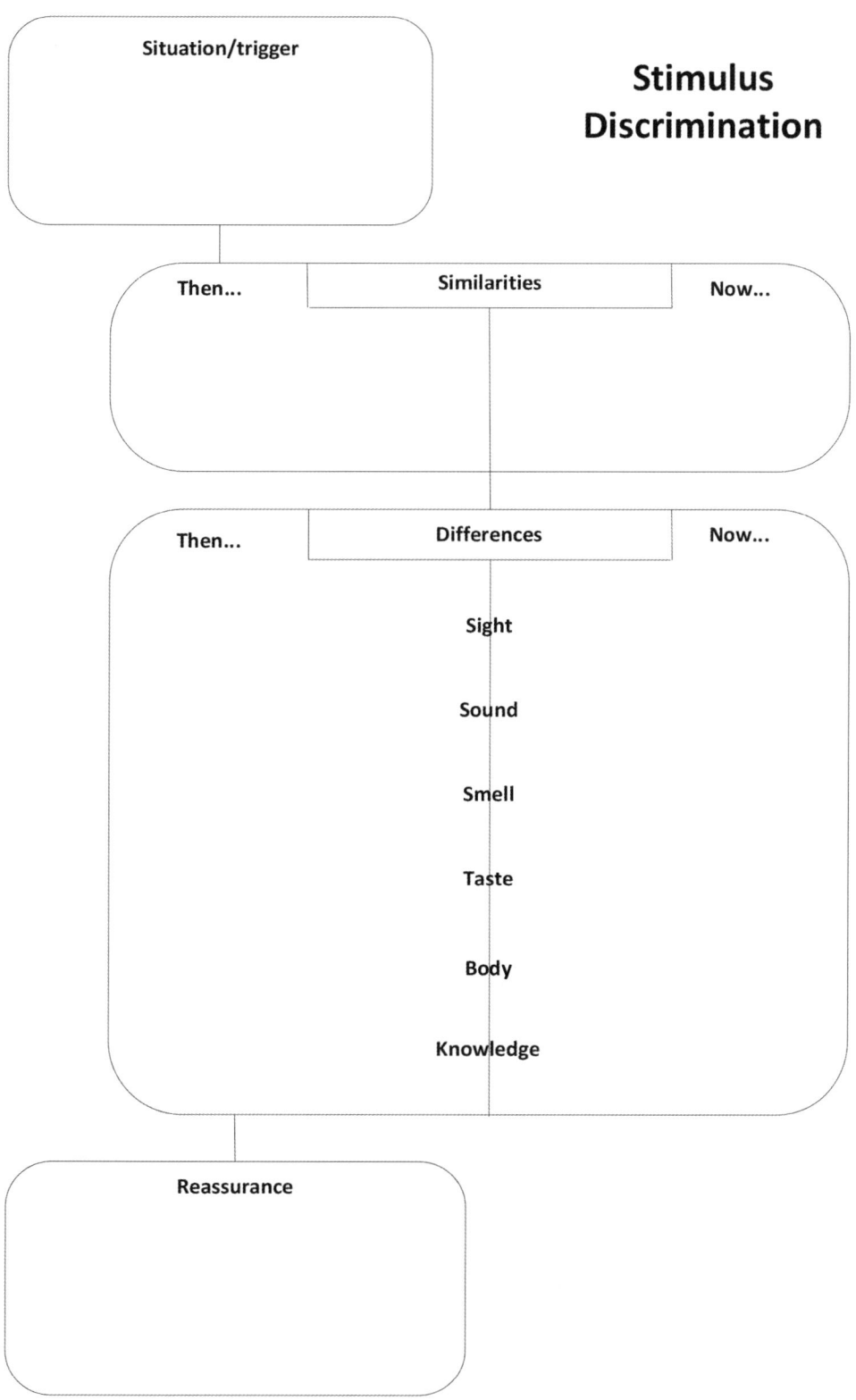

Imagery-Based Exposure

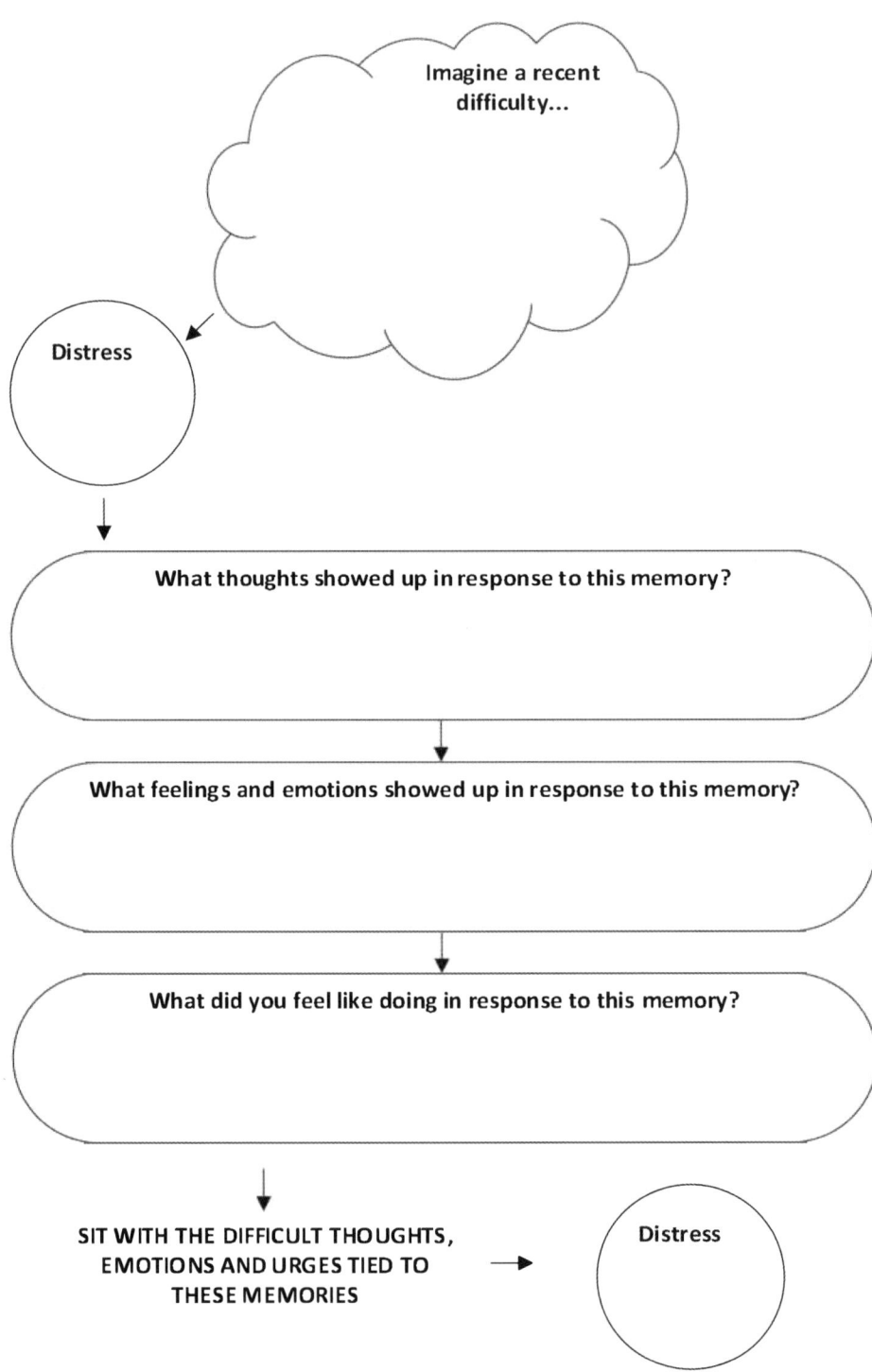

Downward Arrow Model

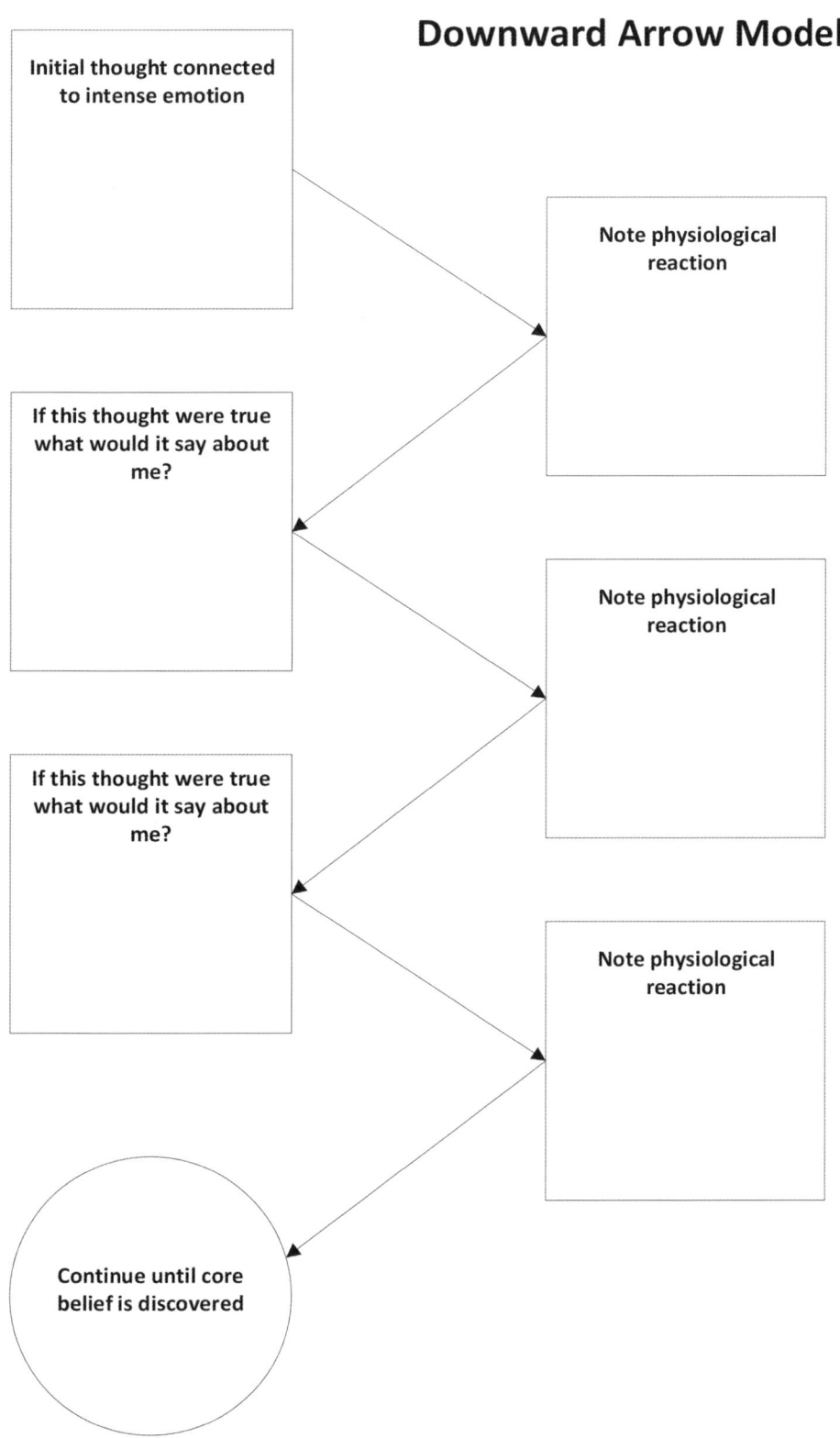

Core Belief Experiment

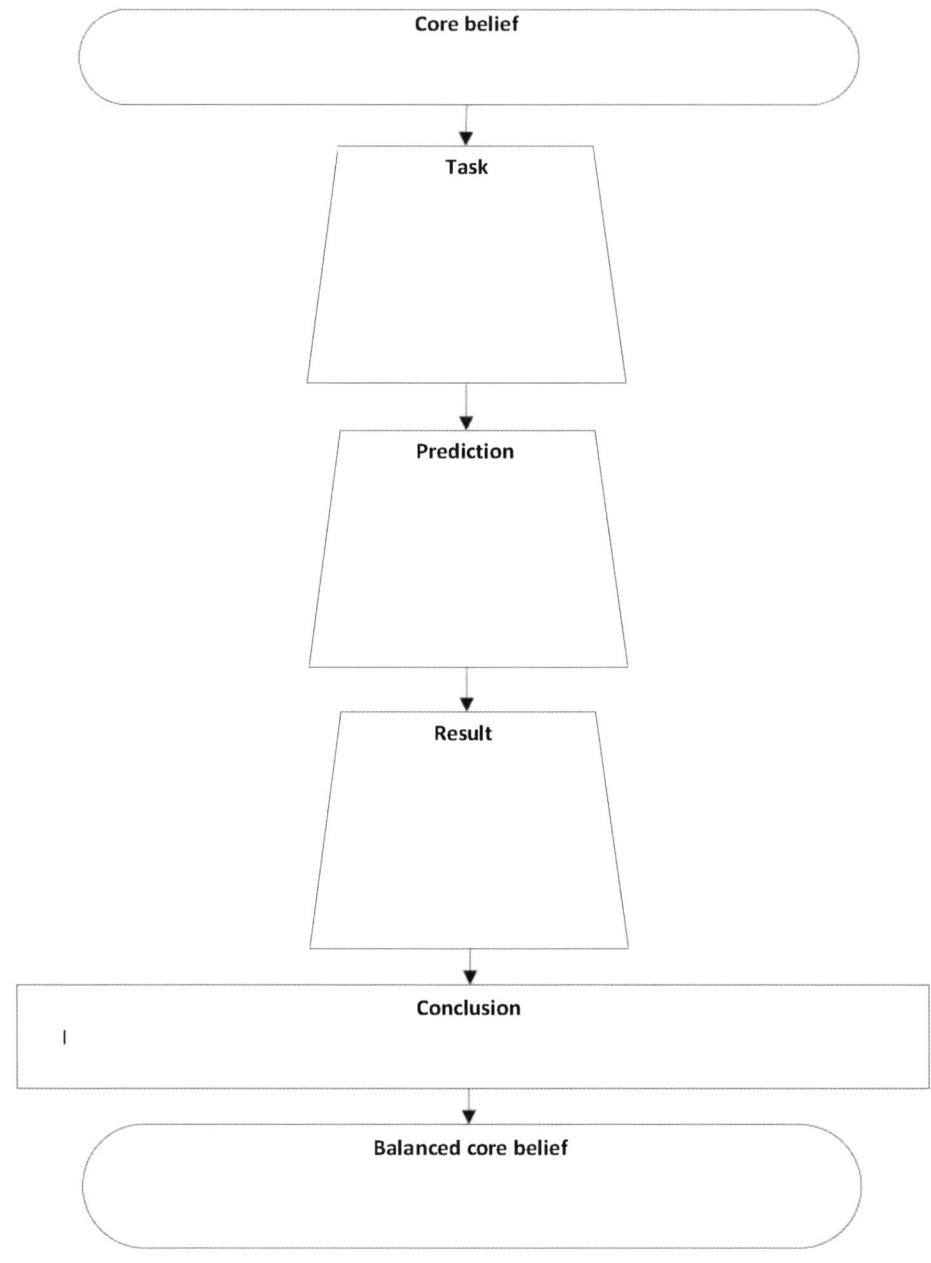

Graded Exposure for Phobias

Date/time	Feared activity	Starting anxiety	Anxiety at end	Reflections	Duration

0 — Target end anxiety

50

100 — Anxiety too high for attempt

OCD Graded Exposure

Situation	Expected anxiety %	What do you predict will happen?	Starting anxiety %	Anxiety at end %	Outcome: what actually happened?	Belief strength %

| The next time I am in _____ situation, |
| I can... |
| |

| The next time I am in _____ situation, |
| I can... |
| |

| The next time I am in _____ situation, |
| I can... |
| |

| The next time I am in _____ situation, |
| I can... |
| |

Coping Cards

> Just because…
>
> doesn't mean…
>
> I know…
>
> is true because…

> Just because…
>
> doesn't mean…
>
> I know…
>
> is true because…

> Just because…
>
> doesn't mean…
>
> I know…
>
> is true because…

> Just because…
>
> doesn't mean…
>
> I know…
>
> is true because…

Cognitive Cue Cards

Acknowledging Needs

Physical needs

Emotional needs

Relationship needs

248 Chapter 7. Interpersonal strategies – Blank worksheets

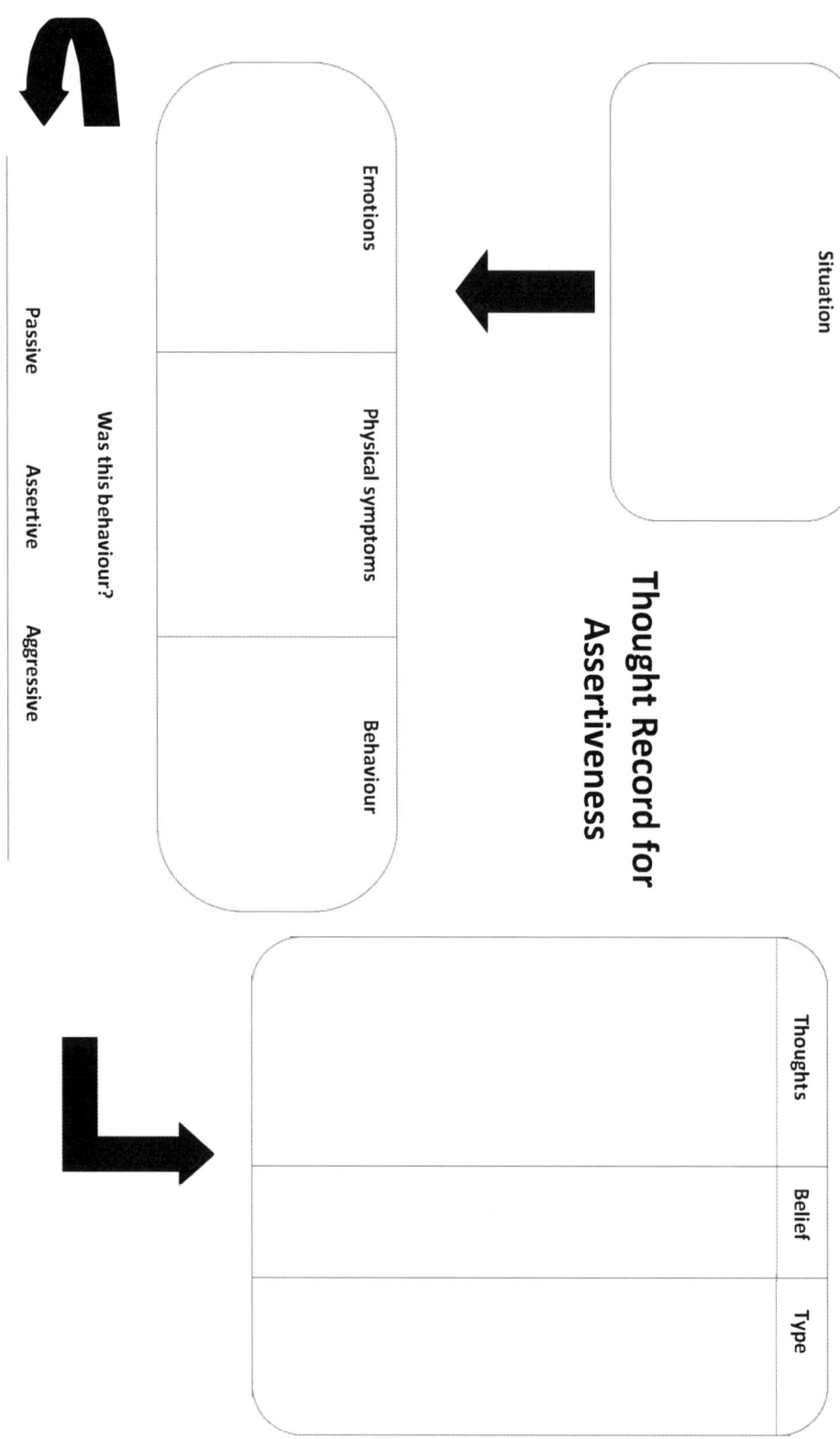

Assertiveness Technique Log

Date/time	Technique used	Situation and how technique was used	Things to remember for next time

Temperature Reading

	Myself	Name_____
Appreciations		
New information		
Puzzles		
Recommendations for change		
Wishes, hopes and dreams		

Circle of Contact

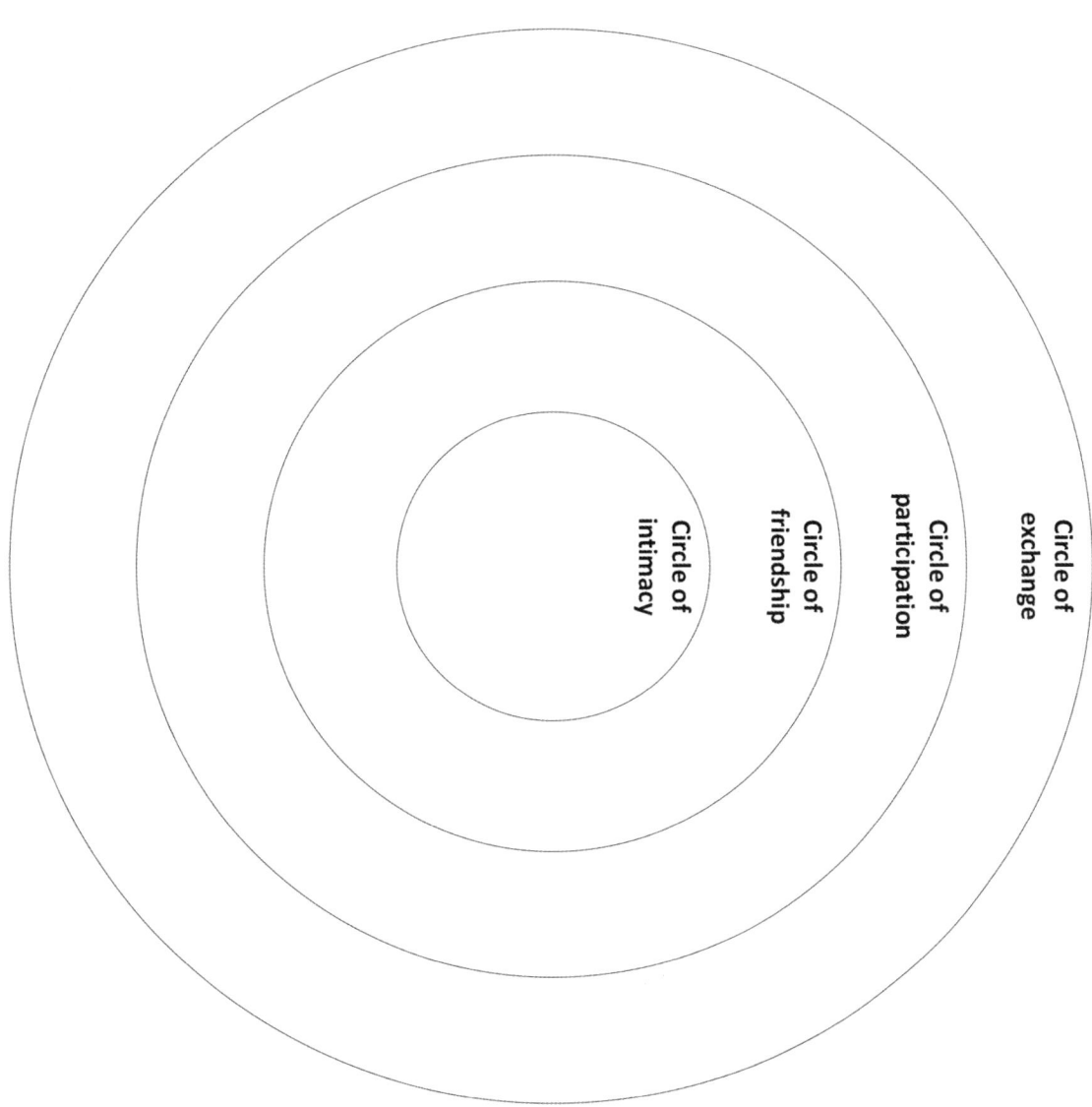

252　Chapter 7. Interpersonal strategies – Blank worksheets

Situation

My son not being at the top of his class

Myself	
	_____ %
Total	100 %

Responsibility Pie

Cycle of Abuse

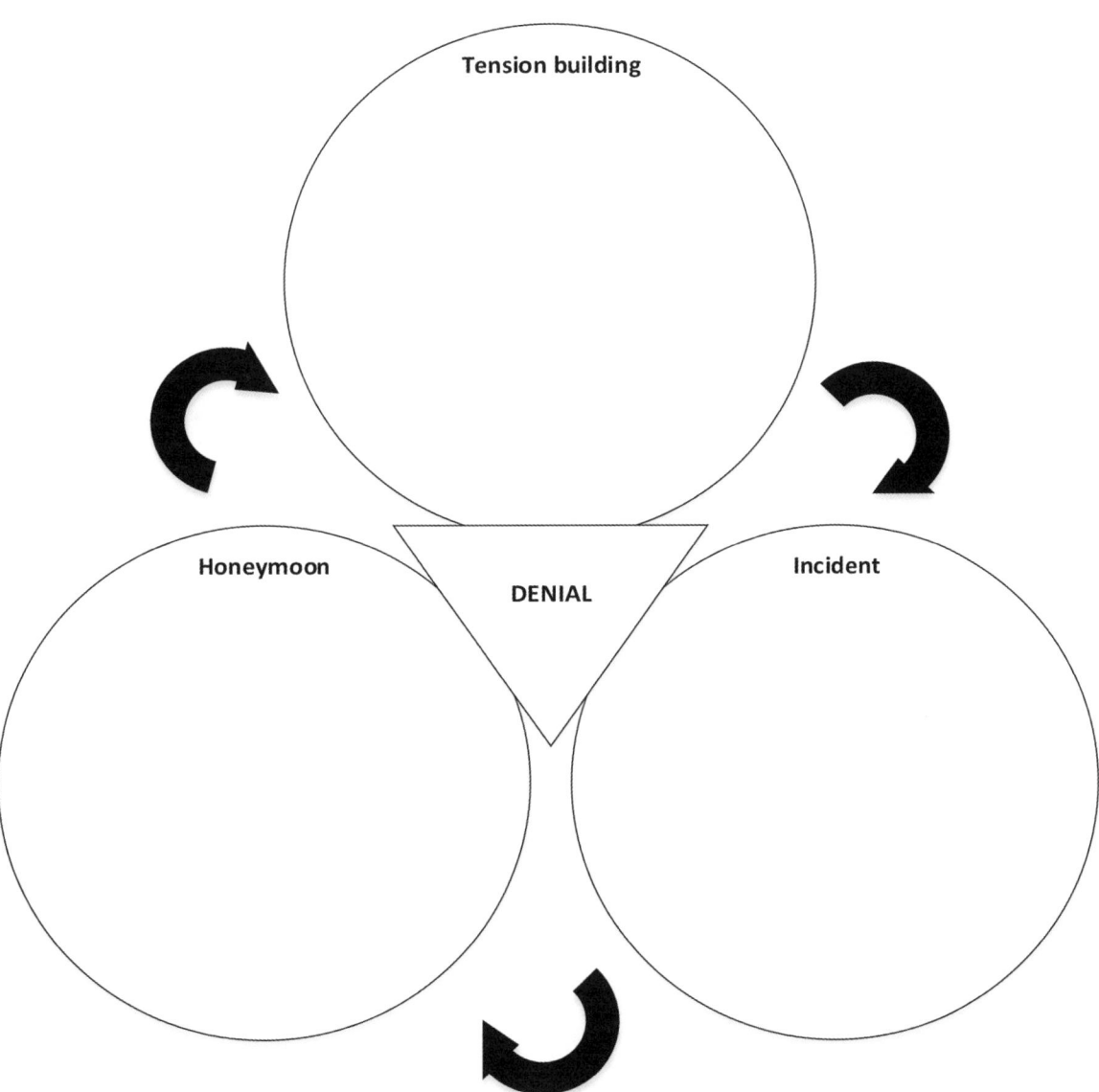

Improvement and Impact Reflection

Work/studies/contribution

Family

Home life

Friendships/relationships

Social life

New Coping Devices Reflection

What therapeutic skills/exercises have proven helpful?

What non-therapeutic activities have proven helpful?

What has helped me put these skills and activities into practice?

Progress not Perfection Charts

Issue	'Perfection'	Where I started	Progress

Issue	'Perfection'	Where I started	Progress

Issue	'Perfection'	Where I started	Progress

Issue	'Perfection'	Where I started	Progress

Issue	'Perfection'	Where I started	Progress

Early Warning Signs

Early warning sign

Early warning sign

Early warning sign

Early warning sign

Action Plan

What are my triggers?	
How can I redirect my attention?	
What tools can I use to resolve the situation?	
How do I keep it SMART?	
How will I know if what I am trying is working?	

Future Plans

How do I build on what I have learned?

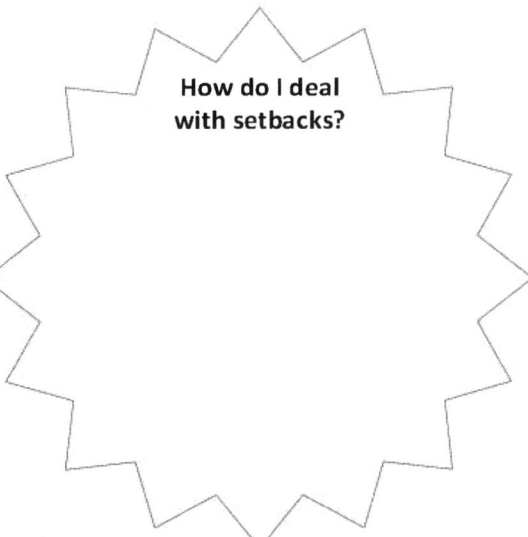

How do I deal with setbacks?

Who can I contact for additional support?

Also by PCCS Books

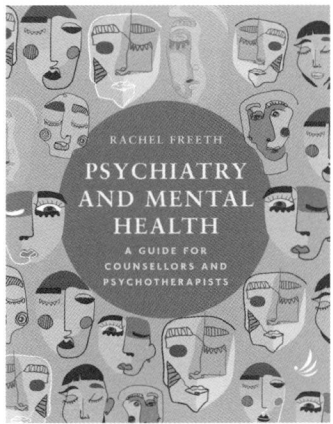

*Psychiatry and Mental Health:
A guide for counsellors and psychotherapists*

Rachel Freeth

(Published 2020, pp. 602)

ISBNs
paperback – 978 1 910919 52 1
epub – 978 1 910919 55 2

Increasingly, counsellors and psychotherapists are working with people who have been diagnosed with a mental disorder and are required to understand and navigate the mental health system. Counselling training rarely covers the fields of psychiatry and mental health diagnoses in detail and there are few reliable resources on which they can draw. This comprehensive guide to psychiatry and the mental health system, written by a psychiatrist and counsellor, aims to fill that gap.

The book is intended for counsellors and psychotherapists but will be helpful to others in the mental health field. It explains the organisation and delivery of mental health services in the UK, the theories and concepts underpinning the practice of psychiatry, the medical model of psychiatric diagnosis and treatment, the main forms of mental disorder, how to work therapeutically with people with a diagnosed mental disorder and how to work with risk of suicide and self-harm. The text is designed to support continuing professional development and training and includes activities, points for learning/discussion and comprehensive references.

Available at discounted price with free UK postage from
www.pccs-books.co.uk